THE NOSTALGIA FACTORY

THE
NOSTALGIA
FACTORY

MEMORY, TIME AND AGEING

DOUWE DRAAISMA

Translated by Liz Waters

YALE UNIVERSITY PRESS
NEW HAVEN AND LONDON

Published with the support of the Dutch Foundation for Literature.

For information about this and other Yale University Press publications, please contact:
U.S. Office: sales.press@yale.edu   www.yalebooks.com
Europe Office: sales@yaleup.co.uk   www.yalebooks.co.uk

Set in Arno by IDSUK (DataConnection) Ltd
Printed in Great Britain by TJ International Ltd, Padstow, Cornwall

Library of Congress Cataloging-in-publication Data

Draaisma, D.
    [Heimweefabriek. English]
    The nostalgia factory: memory, time and ageing / by Douwe Draaisma.
        pages cm
    Translation of the author's De heimweefabriek: geheugen, tijd & ouderdom.
    Includes bibliographical references and index.
    ISBN 978–0–300–18286–6 (alk. paper)
    1. Reminiscing in old age. 2. Reminiscing. 3. Autobiographical memory.
    4. Memory—Age factors. I. Title.
    BF724.85.R45D7313 2013
    155.67'1312—dc23
                                                                    2013016692

A catalogue record for this book is available from the British Library.

10 9 8 7 6 5 4 3 2 1

Contents

Preface

Of all the memories in the Netherlands, which is the oldest? Until the summer of 2005, I would have known the answer. Logic dictated that you had to find the oldest person in the country who was still able to recall early childhood – she turned out to be Hendrikje Schipper of Hoogeveen – and then ask her what was the very first thing she could remember.

Hendrikje came into the world in the summer of 1890, a premature baby weighing barely three pounds. There were no incubators in those days. She survived thanks to her grandmother, who sat by the fire for four weeks holding the child in her lap, in a warm woollen pinafore. It was a chilly summer, it seems. Hendrikje lived to be the oldest person in the Netherlands. When she died she was 115.

Her earliest memory, she said in an interview, concerned that same grandmother. Hendrikje was sitting on a foot stove when her granny handed her a jumble of yarn and made her wind it, endlessly, into a ball. 'You'll have to start over, it's so messily wound.'[1] She was about three at the time, she thinks.

Subtract 3 from 115: the oldest memory in the country was 112 years old and still alive, in a room in a nursing home in Hoogeveen.

But how does such a memory actually live? Did Hendrikje truly remember sitting on the foot stove, in an image laid down in her memory all those years ago? Or had she told the story so often that what she really remembered was the story? For that matter, could it be that as a child she was once told that her granny used to get her to wind yarn into a ball, and the story then transformed itself into a memory? If she does remember the original image rather than a story, whether hers or someone else's, does she perhaps record it afresh every time, so that her earliest memory is really no older than the last time she thought of it?

That is what most psychologists of memory now believe. By recalling something, you lay down a new neural pathway and the next time you apparently remember the same thing, it is actually the most recent pathway that becomes active. Memories, even the oldest, travel in time along with your brain tissue, joined by more and more new impressions. According to this theory, when you think back to your earliest memory a strange kind of contact is made in the neurological circuits that deal with remembering:

the oldest memory becomes the newest for a moment; the first becomes the last.

In a memory that is growing old, other circles seem to close too. One of the characters in *A Tale of Two Cities* by Charles Dickens is Mr Lorry, a man in his late seventies. During a conversation one night he looks back over his life. 'Do the days when you sat at your mother's knee, seem days of very long ago?' someone wants to know. Twenty years earlier he would have answered that they did, says Lorry, but now, in his old age, he has the feeling his life has moved in a circle and he is now closer to the beginning. 'My heart is touched now, by many remembrances that had long fallen asleep.'[2]

Dickens was in his mid-forties when he wrote *A Tale of Two Cities*, so he must have heard about this phenomenon from older people. Günter Grass was the same age as Mr Lorry when he wrote his autobiography *Peeling the Onion*.[3] In an interview with the *Frankfurter Allgemeine Zeitung* a few days before the first German edition appeared, he famously discussed his belated 'confession' that he had served with the Waffen SS, but he also talked about whether it was possible to remember events and experiences of sixty or more years ago at all reliably. As Grass recounted his memories of the great political and artistic debates of the post-war years, one of the journalists, a little sceptical, suddenly asked: 'How far away is all that, when you're almost eighty?' Grass replied: 'It's all very close. If I wanted to say exactly what journey I undertook in 1996, I'd have to consult one of my notebooks. But in old age your childhood grows clearer. The best time to write something autobiographical seems to be connected with your age.'[4] Grass obviously felt that as the years went by, memories of his youth were becoming more vivid.

It is a phenomenon many people say they recognize from personal experience, usually as something that started when they were approaching sixty and has only increased since then. It might be a sudden memory of the face of a person who lived in your street when you were ten, the name of a washing powder that disappeared from the shelves decades ago, something that happened when you were sleeping at a friend's house as a child, or a scene from a book that you read at the age of fourteen. These are memories that emerge unprompted, without any effort on your part to retrieve them; in fact you were not even aware they were there to be retrieved. They seem to have awoken spontaneously from that sleep Mr Lorry talked of. Sometimes they are memories of the 'haven't thought about that for fifty years' kind, and they arrive so crisp and intact that it seems as if they have emerged unspoilt from an ice layer that only now, in old age, is starting to thaw. The name 'permastore' has been proposed for this extremely long-term memory storage, an appropriate metaphor for an experience that makes it seem as if things locked away for many years, inaccessible and frozen, have been released, replete with the scent of their era.

This return of old memories, which psychologists call the 'reminiscence effect', is a mysterious phenomenon. The fact that early memories present themselves spontaneously when we look back seems to contradict what might be called the First Law of Forgetting: the longer ago something happened, the less chance we have of remembering it. No less puzzling is why they seem to emerge again only in old age. They must have been stored away in the memory of the forty-year-old, the fifty-year-old, so why do they surface again when the memory is starting to become truly ancient? It is as if they were under embargo all that time and became available again only after their release date.

The reminiscence effect is at the heart of this book. It has been the subject of much research over the past ten to fifteen years in a field known as the psychology of autobiographical memory. What prompts the return of early memories? When does it start? Do sad memories come back just as readily as happy memories? Is the vivid recollection of experiences early in life a result of biological ripening? Or is it simply that more memorable things happen to us in our youth? Does the effect, once it comes into play, grow stronger with age? Might there be so many early memories because there are so few late memories? These are questions to which we shall return in Chapter 4, 'Reminiscences', but they will arise in several other chapters of this book as well.

Reminiscences have their rightful place in a life story, and they may sometimes actually lead to that story being written down. A good many autobiographies are written by people who were absolutely convinced ten years earlier that they would never so much as contemplate writing about their own lives. The neurologist Oliver Sacks is one of them. As he approached sixty he noticed that memories of his childhood would surface spontaneously. Just like Mr Lorry, he described those memories as if they had been 'asleep' all that time. Once awakened they made their presence felt so powerfully that it was almost as if he had no choice but to write his autobiography, which he called *Uncle Tungsten*. In the conversation I had with him in the autumn of 2005 we discussed the way time speeds up as you get older, how the passage of time can change memories, and how the writing of an autobiography can be a form of psychoanalysis. His reminiscences came through in almost everything he told me as he looked back, especially in his memories of his mother and his desire to be a 'good doctor' in his parents' eyes. In reflecting upon his life he paid little attention to his distinguished career, his books, his honorary doctorates, prestigious appointments and prizes. What occupied him most of all, in his early seventies, was what kind of son he had been.

Oddly, the reminiscence effect increases at an age when the memory as a faculty is starting to decline. Reminiscences are a powerful new element that emerges just when the ability to recall past events is noticeably and measurably weakening. Older people start to have difficulty remembering what they were planning to do. They find it harder to come up with the words they need, and names in particular can easily slip their grasp. Learning things by heart and locating events in time are harder for elderly people. The question is: how do these problems arise, and can anything be done about them? Are there ways of training the memory? Are there things that increase the likelihood of decline?

How can we keep our memories up to scratch? Is forgetfulness simply part of old age? The answers to these questions – as we will see in Chapters 2 and 3 – have consequences not just for the way people deal with their own memories but for the larger issue of where your own personal responsibility for your ability to remember begins and ends.

Much current research into the psychology of memory concerns the reliability of recollections. There are circumstances in which it is essential that a memory matches what actually happened, but there are also places and times – in therapy, when recalling an entire life, in thinking about your parents or writing an autobiography – when you catch your own memory out, as it were, by noticing that certain recollections have changed. This is not a matter of the unreliability of your memory but of having come to see an event or experience in a different light, so that it no longer means what it meant at the time. Older people are more familiar with changes like this than young people, simply because of the asymmetries of life. A sixty-year-old was once twenty, whereas a twenty-year-old has no idea what it is like to be sixty. Which of us would dare to claim that memories of our own upbringing remained precisely the same after we had children? We will look at such memories in Chapter 7, 'Wisdom in hindsight' – because perhaps it is not wisdom that comes with the years but the realization that Kierkegaard was right when he noted in passing, in his journal, that life can only be understood backwards, but it must be lived forwards.

The return of early memories is not always welcome. In old age, reminiscences can induce feelings of acute homesickness. For his book *Cruel Paradise. Life stories of Dutch emigrants*, Hylke Speerstra spoke to people from the Dutch province of Friesland who emigrated shortly after the Second World War.[5] They moved to Canada, America, Australia or New Zealand with the help of the three main emigration agencies in the Netherlands. Travelling out to find them, Speerstra discovered that homesickness can strike twice, shortly after arrival in the new country and again forty or fifty years later when, at the age of seventy or eighty, emigrants found themselves dreaming in the Frisian language and often thinking about the people and places they had parted from half a century ago. In their memory, as in Mr Lorry's, a circle seems to close. They are now older than the parents who watched them depart and they feel more keenly than ever the grief of those left behind. It is not true that time heals all wounds.

CHAPTER ONE

The longest stage

It is no easy thing to tell a person openly that he or she is old. Other people are old, even if they happen to be contemporaries of yours. And if you say of people that they are old, then it will inevitably be because of some deficiency or failing. A person has difficulty walking, fails to follow the conversation properly, cannot stand any commotion – you can tell that person is getting old. You will never hear anyone remark: 'He said such wise things this evening; he's really beginning to get old.' There are plenty of sayings about the wisdom of age and the understanding that comes with the years, but the cold realities of everyday speech indicate that we feel being old means something is not quite right.

This ambivalent attitude to age is evident in magazines for elderly people. Even before opening them you will notice that the titles avoid any mention of old age. They are called things like *Midi* or *Plus*. On the inside pages elderly people are not altogether absent, but they do tend to be fairly young. To judge by the articles, old age (a term consistently avoided) is a period of assiduous sport and travel, of wintering in warm countries, wine-tasting, and taking courses on French Impressionism. It must be the jolliest stage of life too, since those youthful elderly people are all smiles, whether they are on a museum tour or lifting their mountain bikes onto car racks.

The advertisements tell a different story about old age. Readers can request no-obligation estimates for stair lifts ('Move house? Never! But mind you, those stairs . . .'). They are encouraged to visit the optician or to book themselves in for a 'preventative scan'. Leafing through a random issue of the English magazine *Saga* (May 2013), for every travel advertisement inviting elderly readers to enjoy the majesty of the Norwegian fjords or the golf courses on the Isle of Man ('bring your driver'), there are two that refer to health – or, rather, its decline. They include adverts for hearing aids, vitamin and mineral supplements, walk-in baths, pain relief ('gardening made easier'), remedies for restless legs, shoes for those suffering sensitive bunions, denture problems, tinnitus, insomnia, sluggish digestion, night cramps and osteoporosis. The right-hand editorial pages radiate vitality and lust for life, reporting how the elderly are in touch with the modern day ('silver gamers are grabbing the controller') or exploring 'the last wild places'. The left-hand advertising pages offer recliner chairs and 'positional relief from aching joints'. In magazines like these the contrast is stark: senior citizens romp about on a foreign tideline, but the free gift on offer to new subscribers is a blood-pressure monitor.

Even this story, a narrative of decline, deterioration and the loss of vitality, is told in ambiguous terms. The advertisements feature models who must be at least a generation too young for the ailments depicted. Sitting on the stair lift is a man of about forty who in real life probably takes the stairs two at a time – no wonder he is smiling. Riser-recliner chairs suggest a time of life when every seat offered is eyed sceptically with a view to whether you will ever get up from it again, but in the advert the woman sitting in the chair is perhaps in her mid-thirties. It is as if she is trying out her grandmother's chair just for fun. The discomforts of age, in other words, are associated with all kinds of things, but not with age.

Being old, visibly old, is something the reader must be spared wherever possible, even if that reader is old. Our everyday language and the way we imagine 'the third age' – to pick another of the countless euphemisms – points more to repudiation and distancing than to acceptance. It seems we have difficulty valuing old age on its own terms.

Anyone who believes that this is a phenomenon of our time or of the generations now living is mistaken. The notion of old age as a valuable phase of life, characterized by wisdom and ripeness of insight, has always been drowned out by its opposite: old age as a time of decline, sickness and insanity. In the early fourteenth century, Dante wrote of a old age as ship gradually lowering sail as it approaches harbour, a serene image of a destination and of acceptance. But that same century produced hundreds of satires, caricatures, proverbs and stories about the vanity and greed of elderly people. These were often explicit, but sometimes they could be rather more subtle, such as when virtues like moderation and generosity were symbolized by beautiful young women, and sins such as avarice and conceit by ugly old men. Young and beautiful have always been seen as a natural pair, as have old and ugly. Or old and loquacious. In one of the Greek myths, Eos, goddess of dawn, uses flattery to persuade Zeus to grant her lover Tithonus eternal life. It is a dubious gift, as Eos quickly realizes; instead of eternal life she ought to have asked for eternal youth. Now Tithonus is increasingly ancient, his gait is unsteady, and worst of all he talks her ear off. Eventually she can think of no other solution but to turn him into a cricket – and so the myth explains the endless chirruping of crickets. Historians who have studied depictions of old age in earlier times write that our notion that older people were treated with more respect in some indefinable bygone era itself goes back a very long way.[1]

Research into the history of old age has corrected other long-established beliefs, one being that until the twentieth century, when average life expectancy was only just over forty, there were hardly any elderly people. Demographic studies demonstrate that the low average was mainly the result of shockingly high infant and child mortality. Once into adulthood, an individual had a good chance of living to be sixty or older. By the eighteenth century, in countries like Britain and France, people in their sixties made up around 10 per cent of the population. The very elderly were rare, but they were always around.

Nor is it true that 'in the past' elderly people were lovingly accepted into their children's families, where they helped to look after their grandchildren. Here demography tells a grimmer story. That same high child mortality that reduced life expectancy meant that in eighteenth-century Europe, two-thirds of people in their sixties had outlived their children. In the Greco-Roman world the proportions reflect an even harsher reality: a child of ten stood only a 50 per cent chance of having one living grandparent; by the age of twenty that figure had shrunk to less than 1 per cent. Until well into the nineteenth century, families of three generations were rare, more so than families of four generations are now. The stereotype of grandparents spoiling their grandchildren emerged only in the seventeenth century, in the well-to-do classes. Then as now, grandparents preferred to live independently, a wish that was shared by their children – if any were still alive.

In the twentieth century it gradually became normal to be old. Nowadays when someone dies at seventy we say that person died young, and death notices often include the words 'passed away unexpectedly' even when the deceased was in his or her late eighties. The rapid numerical increase in elderly and extremely elderly people has been made highly visible by an explosion in the centenarian population. At the end of 2012 the

Office for National Statistics reported that there were 12,640 centenarians living in the UK. It also stated that the number of Britons reaching the age of 105 or more had nearly doubled in less than a decade: 560 women and 80 men. In the Netherlands, before 1950 there were never more than forty centenarians, yet in 1997 the 1,000 barrier was passed and today more than 700 Dutch people reach the age of a hundred every year. The mayors of the larger cities have quietly abandoned the practice of visiting every new centenarian personally. Despite this huge influx into the eleventh decade, only slightly more than half those who reach 100 will succeed in reaching the age of 101, and of those 101-year-olds, half will have celebrated their final birthday, and so on. The outer edge of the mortality statistics is a perilous place.

In 1900, anyone who had lived for a century had reached double the average life expectancy. Now in the West that average is itself approaching eighty, for women at any rate. Above the age of seventy all those risk factors that can hasten your end – an unhealthy lifestyle, too much alcohol, smoking, obesity – begin to fall away in comparison to that one powerful factor that you can do so reassuringly little about: being male. Among centenarians there are six times as many women as men.

Old age is the longest life stage even for those who do not live to be ninety or a hundred. Baby, infant, toddler, child, adolescent, young adult – you are none of these things for long. If your life takes the course that actuaries have plotted out, you will be old for longer than you were ever young.

In the western world at this point in history, our quarter-century (or more) of old age is a time of paradoxes.[2] Elderly people have never been so healthy. Many illnesses that meant certain death half a century ago can now be cured or even prevented, and many ailments can be eased by drugs or prostheses. 'Old' bodies are better preserved than ever, by a varied diet and by proper care and hygiene. A person of seventy generally looks younger than a sixty-year-old would have done in the generation of his or her grandparents, or than someone who has reached sixty in a part of the world where conditions are more taxing. Yet there has never been an era in which older people have made more effort, with cosmetics or in some cases even surgery, to look as young as possible.

A second paradox has to do with work and pensions. Whether and when a person retired from work was for centuries a personal matter, a decision that depended on health, family circumstances and financial resources. Pensions and annuities started to become available towards the end of the nineteenth century, but even then only gradually, and only for certain occupational groups. State old-age pensions became a universal right no earlier than the mid-twentieth century in most Western countries. In the 1950s and 1960s they were paid out to people who had worked for many years, perhaps from the age of twelve or thirteen, in jobs that took a significant toll on their bodies. Those reaching pensionable age in recent years, born in the 1940s, started work later, usually in much less physically demanding jobs. For the baby boomers now beginning to draw their pensions it is true to say that the distance from the start to the end of a working life has never been so short. The paradox here is that the 'standard' retirement age (sixty-five in many Western countries) introduced a clear boundary precisely at a time when there was less reason for it than ever. Moreover, it represents not just a right but a duty: in many countries most people are forced to leave work on reaching 'retirement age'. There is no justification at all for this sudden, blanket withdrawal from the process of earning a living. Physically demanding jobs have been made far easier by machinery, and the decline of mental faculties in old age is a slow and gradual process that certainly does not warrant a fixed and compulsory cut-off point. Perhaps the credit crunch and dwindling pension funds will help to reverse this situation. The ONS reported that by the end of 2012 nearly a million pensioners were still – or again – working. In the UK, as elsewhere, dropping annuities may force us to rethink the compulsory nature of retirement legislation.

Lastly there is the paradox that in many lives 'old' is the longest epoch, with the fewest gradations within it. Sometimes we distinguish between young and old senior citizens (another euphemism), or between the third and fourth age, but generally we make no attempt to identify distinct phases and stages. Here too language discloses something about our general image of old age: it is a static period, without progress or variation, in which life comes to a standstill.

No matter how many vigorous, healthy and active elderly people we see around us, in developing a perspective on old age we still adhere quite closely to the image drawn or painted in the

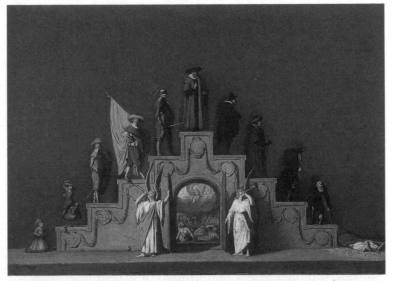

Fig. 1 The 'Ages of Man', *Die Lebenstreppe* (Haarlem, seventeenth-century).

sixteenth and seventeenth centuries as the 'Staircase of Life' or 'Ages of Man'.[3] For symmetry's sake the ages of man were depicted on this staircase as adding up to an even number of years, usually eighty or a hundred, so that the forty- or fifty-year-old would stand at the top. Sometimes the steps were inscribed with mottos or religious poetry, sometimes each age had its own symbolic creature: the eagle and the bull for those aged twenty and thirty, the lion or the sly fox at fifty, the domestic dog for the seventy-year-old and at eighty a cat snoozing in front of the fire. Old age was sometimes symbolized by an owl, but more frequently by a goose or a donkey.[4]

The 'Ages of Man' painted by an anonymous master in about 1680 leaves no room for doubt about how old age was perceived at that time. All the light has been reserved for the first half of life. The colourful flags, plumes, cloaks and sashes give the years of ascent a look of joy that is lacking on the right. On the left side even the angel is more festively clad. No light shines on the years of descent. After the age of fifty we feel our way to our end through the half-darkness, drably dressed.

A second contrast lies in the fact that the first half of life is depicted as a time of change and variety. The young man of twenty with a hawk on his wrist no longer resembles the boy of ten astride his goat; the forty-year-old is absorbed in soldiering and is no longer the *bon vivant* he was at thirty, while the man of fifty, an admonishing finger raised, has new responsibilities as well. Each decade has a character of its own. The descent, by contrast, is of depressing uniformity. All that distinguishes the eighty-year-old from the seventy-year-old is a more pronounced stoop. There is increasing effort and infirmity, walking sticks are needed and eventually crutches, but aside from that an old man is simply an old man, whether aged sixty, seventy, eighty or ninety. Only the centenarian does something novel: he dies.

There is a detail one might easily overlook. The infant, the boy, the young man, the adult, the mature fifty-year-old: they all have their eyes fixed on the world. Viewing the picture, we have the feeling they are answering our gaze; they look back at us, there is contact, they still belong with us in our world. The old men have turned away. They make their descent absorbed in themselves, as if expecting nothing more of life or of company. The man of thirty and the man of seventy are in symmetrical positions in the painting, but the contrast could not be greater. Thirty stands proudly hand on hip, eager to be seen; seventy seems to want nothing more than to be allowed to continue his arduous descent quietly and unnoticed. His gait speaks of deficit and loss. He requires no spectators.

Elderly people today have no lack of an audience – in fact, almost the opposite. Help rushes from all sides. There is great concern for their welfare. It helps that old and poor are no longer two sides of the same coin, as they were for so long. Until the middle of the twentieth century, leaving your job meant the loss of all income, which in the absence of considerable personal assets led to dependence on family, charity or austere public provision. Now elderly people have their own incomes and often savings on top. They have become players in a market.

In this respect too, magazines aimed at the elderly are notable for their ambiguity. On the one hand there is a recognition that old age is a time of increasing infirmity. The second largest category of advertisements capitalizes on this, since an impressive amount of technology has been developed to cater to the physical well-being of elderly people. An 'Ages of Man' painted in our own time would feature not sticks and crutches but sophisticated walking frames and mobility scooters. On the other hand elderly people are welcomed as players in an even larger market: the travel industry. The biggest advertising category in their magazines exhorts the elderly to go on outings, journeys, safaris, city trips, culinary excursions, weekends away, spa visits, walking holidays, art tours, cruises, and to get out and about in all kinds of other ways. Becoming less mobile therefore goes hand in hand with increased mobility. As symbols of old age the crutches, the dog, or the cat snoozing by the fire are outdated. A greater desire to travel balances out the image of the elderly looking inwards, having apparently lost interest in the world. Old people nowadays explore the distant and the exotic.

How about their mental state? The unknown master who painted the man of sixty as having turned away from the world must surely have been trying to express a sense that old age should be a time of repentance; psychological well-being was associated with contemplation of the life that was coming to an end and with timely preparation for death. Below the staircase, a scene depicting the Last Judgment is visible to the viewer throughout. In modern, secular times, a healthy mental state is more likely to be explained as the result of an active lifestyle, a satisfying social life, and intact intellectual and psychological faculties. Some elements may be missing or unsatisfactory, but in that case they need attending to. The market comes into play here as well. The threat of loneliness can be held at bay by special outings for singles and by dating agencies for the elderly. Levels of intellectual capacity are monitored. Should powers of concentration diminish noticeably and the ability to process large amounts of information simultaneously start to falter, then action must be undertaken to reverse the process of decline. Growing old successfully, we are led to believe, demands effort, training, upkeep and indeed expenditure, because everything needed to achieve it is on offer for a price. Just as no one any longer has to accept a deterioration in hearing or eyesight, no one has to accept a decline in intellect, or a weakening of memory.

CHAPTER TWO

Forgetful

Beneath the ascent and descent of the 'Ages of Man' we could trace a curve showing what is known in developmental psychology as the 'parabolic pattern'. This refers to the notion that the time between babyhood and early adulthood is marked by a growth and refinement of our mental and cognitive skills, which takes place in a rapid succession of stages and sensitive periods. The curve showing this pattern is said to reach a peak, after which those same skills, each at its own pace, decline and deteriorate. This perspective on development, the declining part at least, has been superseded of late: most of our cognitive powers remain unimpaired for the rest of our lives.

This does not mean that there are no infirmities of age. Our powers of concentration decline somewhat, the capacity of the working memory reduces and the pace at which new information is processed slows, especially if there is a great deal of it at the same time. Memory problems have a tendency to increase as the years go by. After the age of fifty we fight a dogged battle with forgetting – not for the first time, since this is something we do all our lives, but we tend to be defeated more often.

You might recognize yourself in the following profile. More and more frequently you think to yourself, 'I mustn't forget to . . .', only to realize afterwards that you did forget. You are gradually starting to acknowledge a newly acquired habit of losing track of what you were intending to do, so you start making sure you do things immediately, as far as possible, since that means you will not have time to forget about them. You put that book you want to return to your friend tonight into your bag right away, for example, but then when you get home . . .

Our memory for planned actions, or 'prospective memory', deteriorates noticeably as we get older. This can be confusing precisely because the effect is so similar to that of a trait of which many people are aware all their lives: the absent-mindedness that makes them forget what they came to do, where they were going, or what was supposed to happen next. The difference is that whereas you used to forget your plans because your thoughts were elsewhere, now you have the feeling your thoughts were not elsewhere at all, at least not that you can recall, yet still the plan has vanished into thin air.

Prospective memory has been the subject of much research over the past fifteen years.[1] In experiments in which participants were asked to complete a task that required considerable concentration, while at the same time remembering that they had been instructed to interrupt that task briefly at a specific time to carry out another assignment, older people encountered more problems than younger people. In an experiment no serious consequences ensue, but it may be a different matter in daily life when we need to remember to turn off the oven in half an hour's time, to take medication promptly or to double-lock the door at night.

It is our prospective memory that enables us – or should enable us – to remind ourselves about future actions. In that sense it differs from the type of memory in which past events are stored. Ordinary memories can point to a great diversity of things: people, places, events, actions. Prospective memory contains just one category, planned actions, and they are particularly difficult to retain. An action that has taken place is stored away with all kinds of associations: where it happened, who was present, how it went. With future actions those associations are absent, and because associations function as paths that lead us to memories, our plans and intentions can easily slip our grasp.

The fact that older people find it harder to remember intentions seems above all to be a problem of imprinting. The elderly find it more difficult to store information effectively, especially if that information is as lacking in associations as something that has yet to happen. That same problem of imprinting explains why older people are more likely to forget whether or not they have actually done whatever it was they have kept telling themselves 'I mustn't forget to do'. Like the intention, the act itself is less likely to be properly stored by older people, so they more often find themselves having to check whether they really have locked the front door or only planned to do so. Reminders may have little effect or even be counterproductive – another consequence of the declining ability to imprint.[2] The moment you put that book in your bag, you will probably stop thinking about it, convinced you will remember to give it back. That 'I forgot!' on arriving home is partly the result of defective imprinting caused by an over-reliance on reminders. A second problem with reminders, whether they are notes, clues, mnemonics or some other clever device, is that they depend upon the very processes they are intended to reinforce. You need to remember why you wrote that X on your hand. Does it mean you are supposed to ring someone? To pass on a message? Above all you have to make sure the reminder comes to your attention in time. A note in your diary will help only if you remember to look in your diary. When your prospective memory truly begins to fail, it loses track not only of intentions but of the measures you have taken to remind yourself of your intentions.

Problems with prospective memory are a sensitive indicator of a more general decline. Forgetting what you were intending to do is sometimes the first sign of dementia, but fortunately it is relatively rare for that to be the cause. Dementia can certainly express itself in this way, but more commonly problems with prospective memory are part of the general forgetfulness that comes with age. A paradoxical aspect of this particular form of decline is that it affects not so much the past as the future.

A memory problem that older people mention even more frequently is being unable to find the right word. In their conversations they increasingly resort to 'whatsit' and 'thingummy' or long-winded descriptions of what something looks like, where it can be found or what function it serves. There is a paradox here too: the torment is not so much being unable to find the right word as the knowledge that you know it. At home on the sofa you join in with *University Challenge* and know almost all the answers – it is just that you cannot call them to mind. This endows you with a dubious kind of erudition in the eyes of younger family members, who might judge that your astounding reservoir of knowledge of the 'oh yes, I know this' variety is little different from their own complete ignorance. Those young people are mistaken. Experiments show that old people are more likely than young people to experience a state referred to in the psychological literature as a 'feeling-of-knowing'.[3] In tests that ask participants to provide more formal synonyms for certain words – for example, smuggled goods, a riddle, sleeplessness – the participants can respond in one of three ways: know and give the answer, not know the answer, or know the answer but be unable to come up with it. The last is more common among elderly people, but relieved of the pressure of time they usually do arrive at the right answers in the end: contraband, an enigma, insomnia. This feeling-of-knowing often takes the form of a word that is on the tip of your tongue. Again the elderly are more susceptible, and the fact that they can often give a vowel, the first few letters or the number of syllables indicates that the word really is only fractionally beyond their reach. So older people should not let themselves be talked out of the idea that just because they cannot instantly come up with the linguistic term for a word that sounds like the thing it means, or for a change of syntax within a sentence, they nevertheless know more than someone who has never heard of onomatopoeia or an anacoluthon. 'Oh yes knowledge' is knowledge too.

Even worse than not being able to come up with a word is being unable to remember names. As we get older we start to have more difficulty putting a name to a face when we unexpectedly bump into an acquaintance, or at any rate doing so quickly enough so as to still appear polite. Many people find this to be a particularly annoying consequence of a failing memory, since forgetting someone's name is usually associated with an attitude of indifference. In experiments in which the ability of old people to come up with names was compared to that of young people, the difference did not actually turn out to be particularly dramatic.[4] Two groups – one composed of people in their twenties, the other of people in their seventies – were shown photographs of famous figures and asked to say their names as quickly as possible. The younger test participants did better, but their scores were only slightly higher than those of older people. So why is it so difficult to recall names?

Recognition of someone, whether in a photograph or in real life, takes place in three stages, and there is a hierarchical relationship between them.[5] The first is the visual recognition of a face or general profile, the knowledge that this is a person you know. A second stage almost always follows: knowing how you know the person, what he or she does for a living and what kind of relationship exists between the two of you. In a test with famous faces, of those that were recognized, 93 per cent were identified in some way. The third step turned out to be where the problem lay: the transition from knowing who you are looking at to being able to say what the person is called. In a third of cases, older participants failed to come up with the name of a person they knew. The reverse, knowing someone's name but nothing else about them, is very rare. That tricky step from identity to name can be summed up as 'I'll never forget whatshisname'.

The problem with names is that they have no inherent meaning. Someone who introduces himself as a baker immediately prompts all kinds of associations with the baker's trade: getting up early, kneading dough, clouds of flour. Someone whose name is Baker evokes no image at all. Learning names, experiments show, is just as difficult as learning completely random pairs of words such as 'bicycle–flower'. It is this randomness – someone called Baker might equally well be called Butler – that causes so much trouble for an ageing brain. The absence of associations means there are no other routes that lead to the name, so we remember the baker and forget Mr Baker. There is another problem here too. Being unable to think of a person's name has a greater subjective visibility than being unable to think of a word, since in the latter case you can generally substitute a description or synonym without delay, much as you can get through a conversation in a foreign language despite a limited vocabulary. Not so with names. Your acquaintance has only one – the one that you are unable to think of.

Can anything be done? Sadly, no. Most research on the subject has concentrated on the learning of new names. If brain damage occurs, difficulties in dealing with names almost always result, so there is a pressing need to develop tricks for imprinting them.[6] These usually come down to recommending that the patient provide the associations that names lack, for example by imagining that someone called Baker really is a baker, with the flour still in his hair. It is a laborious technique and the results are meagre, often measurable in experiments that involve presenting people with photographs but not in daily life. Besides, association tricks of this kind carry risks of their own. Mr Baker would probably prefer you to be unable to think of his name than to greet him with: 'Good morning Mr Cook. How are you today?'

When you are elderly, the problem normally lies not so much in learning new names as in quickly calling to mind names you already know. You have been addressing that woman as Mary for thirty years, you know her name perfectly well, it is just that you cannot come up with it right now. Sometimes it helps to have a quick run through the alphabet, in the hope that her initial will pull the rest of her name along behind it, but doing so when you need all your concentration to deal with the uncomfortable situation that has arisen creates a sense of stress that pushes the name further away than ever.

Relax. That is the best thing. You need to accept that there is no reason at all to be ashamed of forgetting names; it is a common ailment. Older people know this. They know that instead of saying 'Hello, er . . . Hello, how are you doing?' they can just as easily say 'Good morning. I know you but I simply can't think of your name'. The temporarily nameless acquaintance should resist taking offence. You have not really forgotten her name anyhow; it will come to you as soon as you have said goodbye. You might call it out after her, were it not that you would probably make a rather odd impression if you did.

In every survey looking at memory in older people, difficulties with prospective memory and with remembering words and names are the top three complaints, but other problems trouble them too. Elderly people start to find it harder to put a time to their memories. Is it three weeks or six since we went out for that meal? Was the most recent election last year or two years ago? Memory is not a video camera continually recording the time and date along with the picture and sound. Whether we are young or old, it is always difficult to recall when something happened, but older people make more mistakes in this regard and their errors are generally in one and the same direction.

In dating our memories we look for markers in personal or public life: it was when we were still in our old house; I was working at so-and-so's then; it was before Obama became president. Putting a date to a memory is difficult, but we can often place it before or after something else, and events with a public character can be used in experiments to determine which mistakes people have made when placing memories in time. In a British experiment, nineteen months after Margaret Thatcher unexpectedly stepped down as prime minister, several thousand people were asked how long they thought it was since she left office.[7] People in their teens, twenties or thirties made an accurate estimate more often than elderly people and if they were wrong it was in a forward direction: almost half of them placed the event too close in time to the present. Among people in their sixties and seventies the opposite happened. They tended to think it had occurred more than nineteen months before.

Divergences like these are evidence of a mechanism called 'telescoping', the idea being that a memory whose details are sharp and clear gives the impression of being looked at through a telescope and therefore seems closer. It is an intuitively plausible mechanism, and it has found support in an experiment.[8] Participants were presented with pairs of events that happened close to each other in time, such as the assassination attempt on President Reagan on 30 March 1981 and the shooting of Pope John Paul II less than six weeks later. A year and a half after those events they could remember far more details about the attack on the president (the participants were Americans) than about the attack on the pope, and this affected their estimates of how long ago the two failed assassination attempts occurred. On average they estimated the shooting of Reagan to have been two months later than it actually was, and the shooting of the pope three months earlier. The forward variant of telescoping seems to play tricks on young people in particular, leading them to underestimate the amount of time that has passed since the event in question. Elderly people err in the opposite direction. Their stored memories are no longer as sharp as they used to be, so it seems to them as if the event happened longer ago than it actually did. This reverse telescoping means that elderly people who ask themselves 'How long is it now since the children came round?' tend to make over-estimates that are hard to reconcile with the astonished 'But we saw you just recently!' of their offspring. Parents and children peer at each other through opposite ends of a telescope.

Forgetting what you planned to do, not being able to come up with the right word, finding that names slip your grasp, no longer knowing exactly how long ago something happened – these are all annoying and sometimes embarrassing inconveniences, but they are hardly the four horsemen of the Apocalypse. Separately or in combination, they are part of an increasing forgetfulness that should not be confused with memory loss or early signs of dementia. There is also some comfort in the knowledge that research on memory failures in young people reveals exactly the same problems: they too forget their plans and fail to come up with words and names; in fact the failings are ranked in exactly the same order.

Since 1992 a study has been underway in the Dutch city of Maastricht into the effects of age on cognitive function. Known as the Maastricht Ageing Study or MAAS, and led by psychologist Jelle Jolles, it has already produced a raft of interesting dissertations, including some on the relationship between age and memory. In one survey of around 2,000 normal, healthy people aged between twenty-four and eighty-six, Rudolf Ponds discovered that just over half the oldest group (aged between sixty-nine and eighty-six) said they were forgetful.[9] In a rather younger group (aged fifty-four to sixty-six) the figure was 40 per cent and even in the youngest group (aged twenty-four to thirty-six) it was 30 per cent. Overall, around 40 per cent of people described themselves as forgetful, so the figure for the oldest group was not a great deal higher than the average, but they did differ in the causes to which they ascribed their forgetfulness. Older people attributed it to their age – they were in their seventies or eighties, so no wonder they sometimes forgot things. Young people were more likely to say they led such busy, exciting and interesting lives that they couldn't possibly remember everything.

Perhaps the most striking outcome of MAAS is the discovery that most older people complain of forgetfulness while still believing they have good memories.[10] They regard themselves as having better memories than others of their age, and when asked to assess their own memories in comparison to those of the average twenty-five-year-old they still believe theirs to be better. A powerful stereotype is probably at work here. Many elderly people are convinced that if you were asked to memorize a lot of things as a child, as their generation was in its day, then you will have a well-trained memory. According to this stereotype, young people no longer have to learn anything by heart, so no wonder they have poor memories. Although not a single study has shown that learning facts by rote has a beneficial effect, many elderly people will give it as an explanation, should one be sought, for the superiority of their own memories. Only when asked to compare their memory now with their own memory at the age of twenty-five will they admit that it has declined. The conclusion must be, the authors write with wry amusement, that elderly people believe their own memories have declined over their lifetimes from excellent to fine but are still so good that they outstrip young and old alike.

The reality, Ponds concludes, is that people's assessment of their own forgetfulness bears no relation at all to how good their memory is according to objective tests. Some people complain about a memory that is in fact still working perfectly well, while others perform very poorly in tests yet think they are blessed with good memories. Part of the discrepancy is fairly easy to explain. In a memory test the participant can settle down and concentrate on the job in hand, whether learning a series of words by heart or memorizing as many as possible of the items shown in a photograph. There is only the one task – no stress, no distractions and in most cases no pressure of time. Those are precisely the factors that create the kinds of problems in daily life that make people start to see themselves as 'forgetful'. Perhaps he might have remembered to post his letter if the phone hadn't rung at precisely that moment; perhaps she might know exactly where she put her glasses if her friend hadn't tapped her on the shoulder. People who complain about their memories think back to that letter or to those glasses, and being able to reproduce a list of words without any difficulty is little comfort.

To gain a firmer grasp of this ordinary, everyday forgetfulness, psychologists have compiled lists of questions that allow people to indicate how often and in what circumstances their memories let them down.[11] The lists include situations such as not being able to find something you have put away, not being able to come up with the name of someone you know, forgetting to pass on a message or suddenly being unable to give a password. Unfortunately such lists are problematic in themselves. If their memories really are declining, people will start to forget about all the things they forgot last week. They may still remember they had to search a long time for their glasses yesterday, but the fact that they have forgotten mislaying their diary last week or spending ages two weeks ago walking around nearby streets trying to recall where they parked their car may lead to an under-reporting of memory problems. In fact even in research using tests that reflect everyday uses of memory, such as those that ask people to recount newspaper articles they have just read or remember directions to a place, it becomes clear that the personal impression an individual has of the quality of his or her own memory is unrelated to how well or badly such a memory test might go. It seems complaints about memory are entirely independent of the actual condition of the memory. So where do they originate?

Ponds and Jolles studied a group of fifty people who were worried about their memories and had signed up for memory training.[12] Their average age was just over sixty. Before their training began they took a long series of tests, including three that measured different kinds of performance: visual memory, verbal memory, and everyday memory tasks such as remembering an appointment or a route. They answered questionnaires on the subject of how memory works in general and about their faith in the capacities of their own memories. There were also tests aimed at assessing aspects of their personalities and their moods. The same battery of tests was administered to a group of the same size in which the participants were of the same age and educational level but had not complained of memory problems. The actual performances of the two groups in memory tests differed hardly at all. Only in one task did the first group perform less well than the control group: recalling as many different professions as possible within a minute. Three other differences were far more telling. People with complaints about their memories scored more highly on the test for depression, meaning they more often complained about being gloomy, lacking initiative, having trouble sleeping or feeling listless. They also had higher scores for neuroticism, which meant they were experiencing more stress and anxiety. Lastly, those complaining of memory loss had little faith in their own ability to remember things. That sounds logical to the point of circularity, but in fact, generally speaking, their memories were no worse than those of people in the control group. Their complaints about their memories seemed more attributable to their gloominess and nervousness than to any actual deficiency. This is important. Rather than working on memory skills as such, people who sign up for memory training ought to be helped to work on their faith in their memories. Without that faith, fear of future memory problems can easily become a self-fulfilling prophesy. Attention becomes focused on things that go wrong rather than on things that go well. People who think they have a poor memory and therefore cease to rely on it will sooner or later prove themselves right.

There is something odd about all these worries. They are focused on the current functioning of the memory, on the ability to store new information, on having rapid access to your own vocabulary, on being able to retain what you have heard, read or seen. It is as if you are standing at the door to a warehouse anxiously checking that the latest delivery is being stored away properly. But meanwhile, behind your back, all kinds of things are disappearing from the warehouse. It is steadily emptying in ways that escape your notice. Memory is dependent on brain tissue, which is susceptible to deterioration and decline, so the memories stored in it fade or disappear. Sometimes you notice this happening and realize that something is missing. You may have read many books on a certain subject and start to notice that you have lost a great deal of the knowledge you gained. Or you come across something you wrote twenty years ago – a letter, a diary entry – and so little of the content seems familiar that it strikes you as impossible that you could have written it. More commonly, things are lost without their disappearance ever coming to your attention. They are gone without being missed. This is the forgetting that takes place unseen.

In one of the final fragments of an essay by Dutch author Karel van het Reve, he writes about taking a stroll one night:

The moon shone through the trees and clouds drifted past the moon. I suddenly remembered a song:

Süsser Mond, du gehst so stille

Durch die Abendwolken hin

I was happy that this song had come to me. There was a time when I would have pushed it aside as banal, but now it occurred to me that perhaps the time was approaching when nothing at all would come to me when I saw the moon and the clouds.[13]

That time was indeed approaching. Van het Reve must have sensed that the decline in his memory was more than 'normal' forgetfulness. But by the time it reached the point when no little songs any longer crossed his mind, he will have been oblivious. The association was not made, and that was all. The memory, even when it does not fall prey to dementia, is much like eyesight. If your field of vision, for whatever reason, begins to narrow, the change will pass unnoticed. You will become aware of the effects once you start bumping into things that you would previously have seen, but you will not be able to tell that your visual field is narrowing, because it has no edges. Similarly, you will not spot any holes in your memory. You may notice the effects, suddenly realizing you do not know something you used to know, but there are no detectable empty spaces.

For that reason alone, memory cannot be compared to an archive or a filing cabinet. If something disappears, then what is left magically closes over the vacant space and everything seems as complete as before. You move through your memory by making associations, since that is how memory works, and associations are linked to what is still there; they never lead you to empty places, because empty places have ceased to be associated with anything. The image of a faltering or damaged memory as something with gaps, hiatuses, lacunas, reflects the view of an outsider. Seen from the inside, the memory is always full.

The documentary *Tegen het vergeten* (*Against Forgetting*) by director Tamara Miranda features a certain Mrs de Rode. She is ninety-two and lives in Groningen, in a spacious and comfortable apartment. She has made hundreds of journeys in her life: '370,608 kilometres on 210 flights with 59 different airlines.' On all those trips she kept travel diaries and she still has them, every single one, along with all the tickets for the flights and for places she visited, all the menus and maps, all the postcards and photographs. Everything is archived in the folders and boxes that line the walls of her apartment. On side tables and in cupboards are hundreds of mementos and souvenirs. As she moves through the living room, with difficulty, in a wheelchair – a sad contrast to her former mobility – she can tell a story about everything she picks up: where she bought it, who gave it to her. It is as if her memory has been turned inside out. Everything she sees and takes out of the boxes has its own associations, so her memories are all around her. The viewer becomes aware of a strange, diverse and highly personal archive. It makes sense because of her memories; without them all those objects would become completely meaningless, as she realizes herself. Eventually Mrs de Rode makes plans to move out of her apartment to a room where there is no space for her collection of keepsakes. Most of it will have to go. But how should she approach the task? What can she take with her? A young man comes round with a notebook to help inventory her collection. We see him and Mrs de Rode, side by side, looking at a wall lined with folders. She makes a touching suggestion. She asks the young man whether she could take something out of each folder so that they become a bit thinner and she can take them all with her.

That is not going to work, of course. In the end she decides against moving and a few years later she dies in her own apartment. But her proposal offers a perfect image of what happens in a memory from which recollections have begun to disappear. Whatever may be removed from them, there is still a complete collection of folders. Nothing appears to be missing.

The fact that forgetting wipes away all trace of itself in the ageing brain is perhaps not the only mercy. All kinds of things may disappear, but cognitive functioning is barely affected until the process is far advanced. It becomes harder to learn something quickly by heart, the concentration span grows shorter and the capacity of the working memory is reduced, but all this happens gradually. The memory is still not spectacularly different from that of a young person, and differences between individuals are considerable. There are no circuits that suddenly stop working, no parts of the brain where the lights go out, no connections abruptly broken. There is only a slow decline, caused by an incremental loss of brain tissue. Dante was right:

the sails are gradually lowered, but only as the ship approaches harbour, not out on the open sea.

The curve showing the development and decline of the cognitive functions is more like a transatlantic flight. After departure it is important to gain height quickly, but then the flight continues at the same altitude for a long time. Only after the age of fifty does a gradual descent set in, with the start of a long downward glide. The sharper descent that heralds the landing will not happen for another twenty years, but anyone who has ever been on a transatlantic flight will remember that the reduction in speed at the beginning of the long descent makes it feel as if the pilot is applying the brakes. You look out of the window in some alarm, see nothing but ocean below and think: 'We're heading downwards far too soon! We're nowhere near land yet!' Of course the pilot knows exactly what he is doing and in reality you are hardly losing altitude at all, but the beginning of the descent is unpleasant and disturbing. People of seventy or eighty who are growing a little forgetful think it is natural at their age and they will see it out, but those aged fifty, still hundreds of miles from their destination think: 'If I'm getting so forgetful already, how bad will it be in five or ten years from now?' You can scare a fifty-year-old rigid by saying, aghast: 'You surely can't have forgotten that!'

CHAPTER THREE

The forgetfulness market

How many kinds of memory are there? Most psychologists are satisfied with the answer 'many, very many', but Endel Tulving – a key figure on the editorial boards of specialist journals on the subject of memory – decided to count them. His answer was 256.[1] Tulving began his project almost as a joke, but looking at the whole inventory you find yourself involuntarily impressed by the number of dimensions a memory has. Time is one of them. Storage can last anywhere from milliseconds to a lifetime. In the iconic memory, visual stimuli are retained for a fraction of a second – a very short time but long enough to make us oblivious to the fact that the world disappears completely for a moment whenever we blink. Visual stimuli remain in the working memory long enough to allow us to look to the side yet carry on cycling down the street without incident. Meanwhile, some things we see remain with us all our lives, in the permastore. To stay with visual memory for a moment, it too can be divided up, according, for example, to the type of information stored in it. Our memory for faces is different from, say, our memory for the symbols on road signs or for chess positions. Each of our five senses has specialized memories like these, and they all have their own timescales and content.

The different types of memory obey their own specific sets of laws. One type is accessible to the conscious mind, while another – motor memory, for instance – may be almost entirely unconscious. One is easy to disrupt, while another continues to function even if the brain is seriously damaged. Our memory for smells develops immediately after birth, autobiographical memory only later. For 'flashbulb memories' – for example, the recollection of what we were doing and who we were with when we heard about the attacks of 11 September 2001 – a single event is sufficient, whereas muscular memory retains only those things that have been ingrained by repetition.

Ask psychologists whether it is possible to train the memory and their first reaction will be to repress a sigh. They are thinking about all those different kinds of memory and wondering where to start. But there is a second reason for that sigh. When doctors talk to patients about how to deal with an illness or disorder, they have an extensive repertoire of terms to choose from. They can talk about recovery, healing, improvement, cure, medication, convalescence, therapy or treatment. Sometimes they can offer nothing more than alleviation of the symptoms: pain relief, a reduction in the speed of decline, the prolongation of life. But no matter what approach they take, doctor and patient have a shared vocabulary at their disposal. A subtle language game has developed around illness. Patients who are told that the doctor cannot offer a cure but can relieve their suffering know what to expect. In the psychology of memory this shared vocabulary is lacking. Conversations on the subject of what to do about memory problems are always difficult, since no language game has developed that does justice to the subtlety of the issues involved. An apparently simple question such as whether you can train your memory is one of the most difficult things you can ask a psychologist.

There is a third reason for the psychologist's repressed sigh, but we shall come to that later.

In a recent television advertisement, actress Nicole Kidman sits cosily in the corner of a sofa solving puzzles on a games console. She turns out to be doing Dr Kawashima's Brain Training, which is recommended in those articles about memory and forgetfulness that are a feature of magazines for senior citizens. 'The more quickly and accurately you play, the higher your score – and the lower your memory age. Anyone playing this game for just a few minutes every day will be stimulating their brainpower, creativity and concentration.'[2] The viewer is told that the game is available from toyshops. Her training is obviously beneficial to Nicole Kidman; she looks at her score with satisfaction and concludes that her memory is once again younger than she had feared.

Not all the puzzles seem equally difficult. If 5 December is a Wednesday, what day is 7 December? If a shopper is asked to pay one dollar and hands over five dollars, what change will he be given? You may have to make a word out of spinning letters, such as D, H, A and E, or add up 7 and 3. Slightly more difficult are reading the time from a mirror image of a clock, deciphering two words spoken simultaneously or indicating as quickly as possible which is the larger of two numbers. The promptness of your answers is recorded and you can develop from walking speed (still need lots of practice) through bicycle speed (making progress) and car speed (moving right along) to train speed, jet speed and rocket speed. The highest possible score denotes an ideal memory age of twenty.

Dr Kawashima really does exist. Ryuta Kawashima (born in 1959) is a neuropsychologist who made his breakthrough in his mid-forties in his native Japan with bestsellers about memory training. Googling his name brings up millions of pages. Type the same name into international catalogues of scientific publications, and the numbers are slightly more manageable. From 1994 on, he appears dozens of times as the co-author of articles reporting on studies involving the use of imaging techniques to show which parts of the brain are involved in specific tasks, such as recognizing faces, names or objects, performing arithmetic, reading aloud or making plans. Not one of these studies looks at memory training. In interviews, which can also be found on the internet, Kawashima tends to refer to the sales figures for his brain trainer rather than to any research on the effectiveness of memory training: millions of people buy it, so it must surely help.

Memory training is now taking place on an industrial scale. Hundreds of books on the subject have been published. Magazines for elderly people carry adverts for training programmes, courses and therapies, and their editorials often address memory problems and what can be done about them. Forgetfulness has been discovered as a gap in the market. The help offered from so many different directions – there are herbs, drinks and capsules on offer – seems to reinforce the notion that although anyone can become forgetful, it is your own responsibility not to stay that way, since you can do something about it. Attempting to improve your memory is therefore part of a larger project: 'growing old successfully'. Memory problems are rather like wrinkles. There is no way to avoid getting them, but modern cosmetic surgery is so advanced that they need not be permanent. Therefore you should not have them.

Memory-training manuals have a mantra, one that is short, rhymes, and is familiar to everyone: use it or lose it. If taken to mean 'stop using your memory and it will decline' then it is perfectly true. Neuropsychologist Rudolf Ponds and neurologist Frans Verhey, both of whom have worked for many years at the Memory Outpatients Clinic of the University Medical Centre in Maastricht, write in their carefully nuanced book about forgetfulness in old age that a lack of faith in your own memory can be the start of a vicious circle.[3] Patients – for that is how they quickly come to see themselves – are convinced they can no longer learn anything new ('I really don't need to try that trick now'), so they leave the operation of new electronic devices to the people around them, stop reading books, get others to deal with bills and paperwork, withdraw from social interaction for fear of saying something they have already said, leave it to their partner to make arrangements ('Could you talk to my wife about that?') and end up not even attempting to learn or remember anything. The worst thing you can do to your memory is to stop using it.

But in a great deal of the literature about memory training, 'use it or lose it' is interpreted very differently, implying that the memory resembles a muscle. The customer, participant or patient is invited to believe that the memory can be strengthened and expanded by training, like a muscle. It is no longer a matter of postponing decline but rather of pumping and toning. In that sense, however, the memory is not like a muscle at all.

In all the rhetoric that surrounds memory training, a number of common features stand out. First there are memory miracles, whether produced by nature or by exercise. Time and again we are told about the student who was trained to remember long series of numbers. At the start he could memorize, like most people, no more than about seven digits. This maximum capacity of seven, plus or minus two, applies to other kinds of information as well, such as words or the names of objects. After training, which lasted a total of more than two hundred hours, he proved able to memorize a series of no fewer than eighty digits, which suggests that the memory really does resemble a muscle. But Ponds and Verhey explain that the student did not develop a larger memory capacity as such; rather, he improved his ability to use a memory strategy. The student, who was also a long-distance runner, accustomed himself to converting the numbers he was asked to remember into world record titles at various distances, or into personal bests. He was no longer memorizing separate figures but the order of, and connections between, times that meant something to him. His capabilities were limited to that task; if he was given words or letters to remember instead of numbers, he could not get much further than the usual seven. His storage capacity was the same as ever.

The same limitations apply to the training of other kinds of memory. Starting on 26 September 2009, Ton Sijbrands played blindfold simultaneous draughts, beating his own record by playing on twenty-eight boards at the same time. After forty-one hours and thirty-six minutes he had won eighteen games, agreed to a draw in seven and lost three. He played 'blind' in the sense that while his opponents were sitting at their boards, Sijbrands, elsewhere in the building, had to call up the state of play in his memory before making his next move. Spectators followed his progress on the internet, and although there was little more to see than Sijbrands, deep in thought, sitting at a table, the knowledge that all those positions and their histories were stored in his head made the mere sight of him impressive. Surely Sijbrands' performance amounts to astounding proof that you can train your brain to such an extent that it assumes almost mythical proportions.

Ton Sijbrands has always been the first to deny that he has an extraordinarily good memory: 'I do believe that I have a good memory for things that interest me, such as literature and politics, but my memory for everyday things is awful. If someone asks if this blindfold draughts player has to take a shopping list to the greengrocer, the answer is yes. My memory is highly selective.'[4] Sijbrands has a perfectly ordinary memory, and it obeys the usual rules for remembering and forgetting. He plays the nine possible opening moves in a fixed order, so that board 10 has the same opening as board 1. This helps him to start off a chain of associations of remembered moves. He then tries to introduce as much variation as possible in the way the games develop, since uniformity would place an additional burden on the memory. Another thing that helps is to have good opponents. A logical sequence of moves gives Sijbrands something to hold on to, and the level of his opponents – top-class players – guarantees there will not be too many blunders, which would be hard to remember. He recalls not just the totality of a series of moves but the development of a pattern. Finally, he stores away those patterns by connecting them with patterns already found in his memory, gleaned from a lifetime of playing draughts at Grand Master level.

As with the student and the apparently dramatic increase in his capacity to remember, it is not Sijbrands' memory itself that has improved but his ability to use memory strategies. Even that specific capacity is extremely selective. Although Sijbrands is a good chess player and has been a club champion several times, he cannot play blind chess. After about four moves the pieces begin to dance about in his head. He says he did not actually 'train' his talent for blind draughts; he discovered it as a child, when staying with a friend who was made to turn the light out at a certain time so that they were forced to continue their game in their heads.

This one specialized form of memory that Sijbrands possesses, however impressive, came into being in a way no different from that of an authority on Proust, a birdwatcher, a Bob Dylan fan, a wine expert or any other sort of specialist or enthusiast. It is not produced by 'training' but by the way in which it is used. Specialists create networks of associations that become extremely compressed, so they can easily retain quantities of facts that seem fabulous to the outsider. Were it not for the cohesion provided by that one specialist subject, nobody would be able to remember so much. An impressive memory is a product not of training but of sustained and dedicated use.

A second common feature of literature on the subject of memory training is the argument 'the richer the environment the better the brain'. It is an assertion that almost always refers back to animal studies designed to investigate 'memory enhancement'. The laboratory animals concerned are mostly mice or rats, and the most common approach is to put a control group of rats into cages for a certain length of time while an experimental group of rats spends the same amount of time in an enriched environment, with exercise wheels, games, mazes and whatever else the researchers can devise in the way of variety. The rats in the latter group will have rather more pleasure in their short lives than the others, but they all end up on the dissecting table. It turns out that the brains of the rats from the enriched environment have more neuronal connections, which on the face of it proves that a stimulus-rich environment results in a better, more efficient brain.

What it actually shows is that the growth of the brain is curbed by extremely stimulus-poor surroundings. A bare cage is not a rat's natural environment. The variety of stimuli provided to the other rats makes their lives rather more like life in the wild. The 'better' brains are in fact normal brains, while those of their unhappy fellow rats have been artificially stunted. A wealth of stimuli can help to prevent rats falling behind, but they cannot make a healthy brain better than it is by nature.

Memory-enhancing herbs, or vitamin and mineral supplements are sold based on a similar fallacy. Substances have been identified whose absence from a person's diet can cause memory disorders, such as vitamin B1, a lack of which eventually leads to Korsakoff syndrome, which causes dense amnesia. A shortage of vitamin E can cause memory problems too. But this is not to say that adding vitamins or minerals above normal healthy levels produces a better than normal memory. Making up a shortfall helps; building up a surplus does not.

A third argument aimed at those thinking of trying memory training is again drawn from neurology. It concerns the presumed reserve capacity of the brain. This does not always take the form of caricature, as in advertisements showing Einstein fixing you with a stare and above him the text 'We use only 10 per cent of our brains!', but the idea that parts of our brains are unused and we can improve our memories by engaging this over-capacity seems to fit so well with what many people already believe that it has become an established feature of advertisements for memory training.

The myth has been in circulation for almost a century.[5] The earliest sources for it are self-improvement courses and books published in America in the 1920s. The assertion has gradually evolved since then, through repetition, into something 'everyone knows'. It turns out to have widespread support even among postgraduate students of psychology.[6] When asked for a source, students will say they 'read it somewhere' or 'heard it in a television programme about the brain'. Books that refer to this myth as part of an effort to encourage people to take up memory training have titles like *Build Your Brain Power* (1986) or *How to be Twice as Smart* (1983). Here too, vague sources are mentioned, ranging from 'No less a pundit than Harvard's great psychologist, William James . . .' (*How to Master Your Memory*), 'A basic contention of Soviet physiologists . . .' (*Superlearning*), 'Psychologists have learned in the last ten years . . .' (*Accelerated Learning*) or 'Psychologists and neurobiologists alike agree . . .' (*You're a Better Student Than You Think*).[7] The references can be no more precise than this because no known study has ever demonstrated that we use only 10 per cent of our brains. When scans using imaging technology show that parts of the brain are completely inactive, this indicates diseased or dead tissue, not reserve capacity. As a matter of fact, the notion of redundancy would contradict the 'use it or lose it' principle: brain cells left unused for years will have died long ago.

Sometimes the argument from reserve capacity is derived from studies of brain damage. A famous and well-documented case is that of a Brazilian boy called Nico, described by his doctor Antonio Battro.[8] To put an end to life-threatening epileptic seizures, Nico underwent a 'functional hemispherectomy' at the age of three; the entire temporal lobe was surgically removed and the rest of the tissue on the right side of his brain was cut off from the left hemisphere and from the brain stem by severing the connecting nerves. The 'disconnected' brain areas remained in the skull, but they could no longer send or receive signals. In a child of three the brain weighs on average around 1,100 grams. In Nico's case, 300 grams were removed and another 300 grams made non-functional. As an adult he will have no more than 700 grams of working brain tissue, half the amount that is normal for a grown man.

Battro called his book *Half a Brain is Enough*. When it was published, Nico was eight. He was attending a normal school, and although he had slight motor handicaps, he was in other ways ahead of other boys of his age and no one who met him would ever guess that he was having to make do with half a brain.

Actually, says Battro, that notion of making do is misleading, since all the boy's education and rehabilitation was aimed at making one half of the brain into a complete brain. Nico's case became a study in 'neuroeducation', or how to support a damaged brain with prostheses, exercises and techniques of compensation in such a way that it can perform as many of its normal functions as possible.

The hemisphere that was spared developed a number of compensatory mechanisms. In an intact brain, information from the left side of the visual field of each eye goes to the right half of the brain. In Nico's brain it goes nowhere, but tests with a stereoscope showed that the left hemisphere of his brain was receiving enough information from the right half of the visual field to enable him to perceive depth. Nico is no less able to judge distances than other children. He went through the phases of childhood development at a normal rate or more quickly. He understood earlier than others of the same age that a ball of clay rolled into a sausage shape had not grown any bigger; he showed no hesitation in drawing the level of the liquid in a glass held at an angle as horizontal, and the trees on a hill growing upwards rather than perpendicular to the slope. It seems you can lead a relatively normal life even with half your brain missing. So, you might ask, what is the other half for? Doesn't this mean that we are walking around with a vast over-capacity in our brains? All that plasticity, all that reserve capacity – shouldn't we be making better use of it?

Sadly, that would be the wrong conclusion. The facts come nowhere close to supporting the claim that half a brain can do double its normal amount of work, even in Nico's case. First of all, he was 'fortunate' that the focus of his epilepsy was located in the right half of the brain, or rather that his linguistic functions had already been laid down in the left half. Much research has been carried out on people who have lost large parts of the right hemisphere, but in not a single case did this cause problems with language. If the left hemisphere has to be removed, the consequences are far more drastic, since along with language the capacity for abstract thought is lost. The two halves of the brain are by no means interchangeable.

A second factor in Nico's favour is that he was operated on so young. There is a 'rule' in neurosurgery: the earlier the damage, the more limited the loss. Opinions differ as to how plastic the brain is, but it is clear that the capacity for neuronal improvisation declines with age. The reason is simple. Functions that have already found their place in the brain are lost if that part is damaged, whereas functions that develop later are allocated a place in the brain tissue that is still intact. Brain damage at an early age is rather like the sudden locking of a room while the interior of the house is still being furnished. It is a shame about the loss of that room, but you simply distribute your belongings around the rest of the building. Brain damage in a rather older person is more like locking a room in a fully furnished and occupied dwelling. Whatever was in that room is lost. A blocked blood vessel or a mild stroke in an older brain has very different consequences from the same event in youth.

A brain that is damaged, even one that is getting on in years, may demonstrate an impressive capacity for self-repair. It is as if reconstruction work begins immediately, creating a neural network of replacement bridges, detours and short cuts. This natural recovery can be supported by appropriate therapies. With enough effort – by patients themselves, their therapists and people close to them – many of the lost functions can be restored or compensated for in some way. This is an encouraging thought. But it does not amount to evidence that, in an intact brain, large areas have lain idle for years and can now be developed through 'training'. In evolutionary terms that would be odd. The brain has a folded structure and in places even the folds are folded. This is a consequence of a lack of space. The neocortex grew so quickly in evolutionary terms that it had to be crumpled up, so the notion that we are walking around with a kind of neuronal spare tyre is biologically preposterous.

The curious thing about all these references to an enriched environment, extra stimuli and neuronal over-capacity is that the techniques presented as memory training have nothing to do with a larger or better brain. They demand mental rather than neurological investment. You are asked to learn series of words by heart and then 'hang up' the things you will need to recall later, while drumming mnemonics into your head and becoming accustomed to 'visualizing', so that an image will enable you to retrieve what you are hoping to remember. Before making a speech you are supposed to think of a house and to leave an object in each room that symbolizes a subject, then make sure you remember the route you are meant to take through that imaginary house while delivering the speech. As well as being artificial, many of the techniques recommended are laborious, such as thinking of associations for new names or remembering the advice on how to spell the word 'professor': imagine the professor with one Football and two Shoes.[9] (And that is just 'professor'; the instructions for 'parallelogram' are three times as long.) Another book of exercises suggests using the mnemonic 'Sergeant Major Hates Eating Onions' to remember the names of the Great Lakes of the United States from west to east: Superior, Michigan, Huron, Erie, Ontario.[10] Anyone planning to follow all this helpful advice will need to have a pretty good memory to start with. Studies into the effects show that such newly learned memory techniques are hardly ever used in daily life. Ponds and Verhey therefore limit themselves to advice that works in practice and is actually pure common sense: write things down in your diary immediately or make notes on the calendar; put things away in the same place every time as far as possible; pay attention while doing the things you have to do, so that you will be certain you have done them.

Most memory techniques are all but irrelevant to the kinds of forgetfulness identified by scientists in surveys where respondents are asked questions about their memories. It is annoying to be unable to think of an acquaintance's name, but you would have to be fairly desperate to put the names of everyone you know through the mill of invented associations just to be on the safe side. Not being able to think of a word is something we simply cannot help. Memory techniques work relatively well with purely factual information, such as PINs, passwords, or the order in which certain tasks need to be carried out, but those are things you might just as well write down. 'The palest ink is more reliable than the most powerful memory', as Confucius put it. People who bewail their declining memory are not thinking primarily of PINs or even names; they regret being able to tell you so little about a film they saw last week, or that if they put a book aside after ten pages and pick it up again a few days later, they might as well start reading from page one. This is a deterioration that has to do with autobiographical memory and unfortunately there are no memory techniques for that. Much of what is on offer under the heading 'improve your memory' comes down to learning tricks for coping with the effects of decline. Anyone who thinks that such tricks – or Dr Kawashima's puzzles – can actually give them a better memory probably also thinks they would be able to walk better if they used a walking frame.

The mantra 'use it or lose it' is true only in its most restricted sense. There is a convincing amount of research to show that the memory will decline if no longer stimulated. The best way to prevent this is to remain active. People who start withdrawing from engagement in regular activities such as voluntary work, theatre visits or participation in a reading group are actively undermining their own memory. The good news is that social activities are sufficient. They involve all the variety and challenges needed to keep the memory up to scratch.[11] Remaining socially active does not just mean that you have more reason to call upon your memory; it also gives you the opportunity to compare your own memory – and its occasional failings – with others. Sharing your experiences of forgetfulness can have a reassuring effect in itself.

However active your lifestyle, however varied your existence, your memory will gradually decline with age. This is perfectly natural. Anyone who still has the memory of a twenty-year-old at the age of seventy is not entirely normal. For commercial reasons, older people are invited to take a different view. The marketing that has grown up around memory encourages the shifting of forgetfulness from normal to pathological, from something that goes along with growing older to a symptom – because a symptom points to a sickness and therefore to medicines, therapies, training courses, curative herbs, supplements and all those other items for sale in the forgetfulness market. Those who sell into that market want their customers to see themselves as patients.

Behind worries about not being able to come up with a name or occasionally forgetting what you were planning to do lies the fear of something worse. If dementia expresses itself in problems with remembering, then surely forgetting to pass on a message or not knowing where you put your car keys might be the first sign of dementia. Many people who go to see their doctor or visit a memory clinic say they can live with their forgetfulness just as long as it does not presage dementia. Fortunately, most of them can be reassured. The likelihood of dementia increases with age, but for people over sixty-five it is still less than 5 per cent. For those one in twenty – and their loved ones – it is a truly miserable fate, but even in those seeking help with memory problems, the probability of dementia being the cause is not very high.

Increased awareness of Alzheimer's disease and other forms of dementia has created a growing community of people referred to in the literature as the worried well. There are many people in middle age who have a father or mother with Alzheimer's and are so worried about developing the disease themselves that it is already adversely affecting their lives.[12] Clinically speaking they have no symptoms of dementia at all, but they are perpetually on the lookout for the first signs of it. Incidents that anyone else would regard as the result of normal forgetfulness or attribute to absent-mindedness or stress represent to them confirmation that the disease has started to take its toll. Fear of suffering is itself a form of suffering; the prospect of sharing their parents' fate may cause them to slide into depression, and unfortunately the symptoms of depression can have a disastrous effect on the condition of the memory. Statistically speaking, the likelihood of suffering from dementia is not hugely increased if one parent has dementia (from 5 to less than 10 per cent) but the worried well are not reassured by statistics – which after all did not help their parents. Someone who has never seen dementia at close hand may well regard 5 or 10 per cent as a low figure, but those who recall the havoc it wreaked when it struck someone in their family or their circle of friends may be unable to avoid that percentage becoming, as it were, multiplied by their sorrow and anxiety so that a small likelihood becomes a real threat.

There is much reassurance to be derived from insight into the differences between dementia and the forgetfulness of old age.[13] The latter falls within the limits of what is natural and normal, and practically all elderly people suffer from it to some extent. Dementia is a disease. Forgetfulness is annoying and troublesome but does not turn you into an invalid, whereas dementia does. Forgetfulness is limited to the memory, whereas dementia also affects the capacity to do everyday things: to get dressed, to make coffee or to drive a car. People suffering from dementia may look at the clock and realize that they cannot work out what time it is. Or they might stand in the kitchen holding a tin opener unable to remember how to use it to open a tin.

Even where the effects of normal forgetfulness and dementia coincide, at moments when the memory fails, there are in reality always clear differences. People who are forgetful may be unable to remember who has just called them, but not that they were speaking to someone on the phone just now. They may forget to pass on a message, but later they will remember what the message was. They may forget the details of something that happened yesterday, but they are capable of being reminded. A person suffering from dementia has nothing left to be reminded about. The difference can be seen even in the use of mnemonics and other memory tricks. Those with a tendency to forget things will often stick up notes at strategic places. Those with dementia do the same, but they quickly forget what they mean or why they are there. It is all very well to have written 'Ring Carl', but what am I supposed to say to Carl? And anyhow – Carl who? The vast majority of people who turn up at memory clinics give such a detailed account of all the things that have slipped their minds recently that it is clear they have no reason to worry.

When memory problems are indeed attributable to the start of dementia, something begins to happen that seems to prove the memory trainers right after all. A man does the crossword in the newspaper every week. He gets stuck more and more often and eventually stops trying. He always used to enjoy reading books. The people living with him notice that these days he starts them but never finishes. A little while later he gives up reading books altogether, preferring to pick up a newspaper or magazine. He passes over the longer or more difficult articles and gradually it becomes more a matter of turning the pages than of reading. Some time later he might keep picking up the same magazine without seeming to notice that he leafed through it the previous day as well.

Is his memory declining because he makes fewer and fewer demands of it? No, it is the other way around: the limitations of his memory steadily close off fields of activity he used to visit with great pleasure when his memory was still intact. The retreat takes place deceptively slowly, but it is visible to those around him in the books that remain unread, the documentaries that he can no longer follow, the letters that go unanswered. At that point no one wants to hear the cries of the market. Overoptimistic ideas about what you can do to stop the decline in your memory have a shadow side: they encourage the notion that it is people's own fault if their memory fails. This does not hold true for ordinary forgetfulness, and in the early stages of dementia it only adds insult to injury – the third reason for the psychologist's sigh.

CHAPTER FOUR

Reminiscences

In the Spanish novel *Los disparos del cazador* (*The Shots of the Hunter*), Rafael Chirbes introduces his readers to Carlos Ciscar, a former building contractor in Madrid.[1] Ciscar is in his seventies and a widower. His daughter died young and he is estranged from his son. He lives with a faithful servant, Ramón, in a large house that has become increasingly empty. Many of his friends have died, the places where he always liked to spend time have either changed beyond recognition or lost their attraction for him. Since breaking his hip he has had difficulty walking. He needs help in everything he does and he shuffles his way through his daily tasks leaning on Ramón's arm. His days are laborious, quiet and slow.

Ciscar's memory, in painful contrast, is more active and nimble than ever. One recollection after another comes to him, in quick succession, whether he is lying in bed, taking a bath, having his midday meal, sitting in the garden or even just looking around the living room. They pounce on him and he is defenceless; he feels besieged by his own memory. Now that it cannot be very long before the shots of the hunter ring out, his memory is calling up a lifetime's worth of recollections, which will all have to be contemplated and assessed one final time.

We often think of our memories as being at our beck and call, rather like an inner servant, a Ramón we can send off to fetch this recollection or that. But Ciscar realizes that he has completely lost control of his memory. However much he would like to, he cannot recall the sound of his mistress Elena's voice. Of his moments of happiness with his young family, in the time when he lived in a house they built by the sea in Misent, little remains but a few paltry impressions. Sometimes, he thinks, 'it's as if only pain has a memory', since the things he does recall take him back to the cooling of his marriage, his arguments with lovers, the friend he betrayed, the fights with his son, or his wife's illness.

What can he do about his mutinous memory? From time to time he leafs through old photographs. When the children were young he bought a Leica. Their lives were documented in a series of snaps: running in the garden, laughing on the beach, their first communion. But in Ciscar's daydreams the boundary between memories and photographs starts to blur. He thinks to himself: 'I can still see some of the photos before me: the beach nearby, covered in seaweed that's hauled away in wheelbarrows in the late afternoon, the café, which reminds me of the smell of grilled fish, the hammock where Eva lies stretched out with a book in her hand . . .'

'I can still see some of the photos before me' – you might almost overlook the fact that what he is remembering is the photos, not the events they depict. Ciscar took the pictures to buttress his memory when calling up a scene, an event, a story, but what he now remembers are the photos themselves. In his memory, the relationship between photo and recollection has been turned on its head. Ciscar has a sense of ambiguity when he leafs through his photo albums. Placed in chronological order, the photos he took of his children show their two lives, helping him to remember how those lives developed. At the same time he cannot rid himself of all he knows about what was to follow those childhoods. It makes him look at the photos differently, as if something must be visible in those early snaps of the turn their lives were to take. The girl on the beach is no longer just the girl of that time but the daughter who will die; the boy running around is already the son with whom he will lose touch. What the Leica captured and froze has travelled with him through time and it now blends with his memories. Long ago, when he still went hunting, he was attracted by the warmth of freshly killed game, a warmth that meant the animal was still halfway between life and death. In the photos he sometimes feels that same warmth. He carefully runs his thumb over them and for a moment he is with those who are no longer around. More often, though, the photo is already a corpse. His parents lie yellowed in the dresser drawers, his daughter exists only in old photographs, which have not been able to reverse mortality – if anything they serve to underline it. He is still alive, both inside and outside the drawer, Ciscar muses, but 'life outside it is more fragile than life inside. Sometimes, when I look at all these photos I suddenly think they are lying there waiting until all our movements stop, so that they will be left as the only truth.'[2]

What has psychology to say about memories such as these? For a long time it said precious little. Psychologists have a professional preference for questions that will furnish the most precise answers possible, so they need to be able to compare what is recalled with what once entered the memory. Most research focuses on memories of things psychologists themselves have fed into the brain: a series of words, a photograph, a film fragment. What test participants then manage to reproduce can be expressed in numerical terms, as a percentage. But no account has been kept of the events that Ciscar remembers in later life. What he now recalls of his arguments with his son as the boy grew up cannot be set beside a record of all those arguments, if it is even possible to imagine such a thing. No one can check Ciscar's memories for accuracy.

It is only in the past twenty years or so that psychologists have recognized that reliability may not always be the most important thing about memories. Might it not be more to the point that such memories return in old age far more often and far more vividly than during middle age? Or that mood has so much influence on what emerges from the memory? Gloomy and lonely people make a selection from their memories that compounds the gloom – a mechanism that seems to play tricks on Ciscar. Again, it is not a question of whether those recollections are reliable; what matters is the fact that such forces are at work in the memory.[3]

Psychological research into the reminiscence effect often makes use of cue words. Participants are shown a word – 'circus', say – and asked to talk about a memory the word conjures up. Attempts are then made to date that memory. Anyone who performs this experiment with elderly people and arranges their

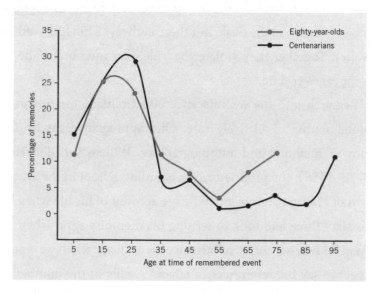

Fig. 2 The reminiscence effect in people aged eighty and one hundred.

memories according to the participant's age will produce a curve with a characteristic shape (see Figure 2).[4] Most people's earliest memories date back to the age of three or four. Then the curve rises steeply, reaching a peak at around the age of twenty before falling back, flattening out and sweeping up again at the end. That final flip upwards results from what is known as a recency effect: if grandparents have been to the circus recently with their grandchildren, then there is a good chance they will talk about their memories of that. If test participants are asked to describe four particularly vivid memories, things they would definitely include in an autobiography were they ever to write one, then that final upward flip disappears to be replaced by an even higher peak at about twenty years old.[5] This 'reminiscence bump' in the curve has intrigued memory psychologists for the past twenty years or so. The width of the bump varies somewhat, as does the precise location of the peak, but there is always a hill followed by a valley. Together they violate the 'rule' that memories fade or disappear over time.

Research into the reminiscence effect outside of an experimental setting is relatively rare. One approach might be the study of memoirs and autobiographies. Willem van den Hull (1778–1858), the proprietor of a boarding school in the Dutch town of Haarlem, wrote an 800-page account of his life when he was sixty-three and took to writing his memoirs again when he was in his mid-seventies, in other words at an age when we would expect to see the reminiscence effect.[6] A tally of the number of pages he devoted to the various phases of his life indicates that for the period from the age of four to the age of fifteen he devoted an average of fourteen pages to each year, and this increased to an average of sixteen pages for the years up to and including the age of twenty-seven. In writing about his thirties the average fell to ten pages. Only a passionate but unrequited love – 'In the entire universe I saw no one but Lina' – raised the number slightly, but after that it declined to less than four pages per year for a period of eighteen years, between the ages of fifty-four and seventy-two. A graph of the number of pages he filled for each year of life would precisely coincide with graphs for test participants who describe the memories they would want to include in an autobiography. A rather larger study along these lines would be able to test whether elderly authors (those in their seventies) use proportionately more space in their autobiographies for memories from the reminiscence period than authors in their fifties.

Sometimes even in autobiographies that are limited to the first half of a life we can see a 'bulge' around the reminiscence period. In his autobiography *Peeling the Onion*, Günter Grass describes roughly the first thirty years of his life.[7] He does not have a great deal to say about his first ten or fifteen years. By page 75 the protagonist is already sixteen. But then it takes until page 116 before he is seventeen and until page 198 – the best part of another hundred pages – before he is eighteen. Not until page 294 does he reach the age of twenty-one. This sideways expansion of time, as Dutch writer A.F.Th. van der Heijden describes it, coincides to a great degree with the Second World War, but also with his formative years. After that the ten years up to the age of thirty-two take less than 130 pages, in shorter and shorter portions, culminating in the statement that he has no desire to tell the rest. *Peeling the Onion*, in other words, has the typical reminiscence structure that betrays an author's advanced age.

Over the past twenty years, various explanations of the reminiscence effect have been proposed. They each seem to present different findings and results, but they do fall roughly into two camps. To put it rather cryptically, one kind of explanation seeks answers in the nature of the memory, the other in the type of recollection.

Biologically-oriented explanations fall into the first of the two categories. They reflect the parabolic pattern of ripening and decay. In childhood and early adulthood the cognitive faculties, such as memory and concentration, reach an optimum. This is the period in which, to stick with the jargon, the species reproduces itself. The ripening of the brain is attuned to our reproductive needs. In the period when partners are sought and children arrive, when parents are responsible for nourishment and upbringing, the brain is in an optimal condition. The argument goes that even now that we are no longer hunter-gatherers, the brain, because of the way it has evolved, continues to produce a reminiscence bump, so our experiences in that period have a far better chance of being stored away properly than things that happen to us later in life. Because of their more effective storage, these are the memories that are more often picked up later, which gives them a further advantage. The experiences of forty-year-olds, with their already rather timeworn faculties, have less prospect of being laid down as vivid memories.

From a biological perspective, consideration has also been given to why such a phenomenon as the reminiscence effect exists. What is its function? In evolutionary psychology this question is part of the larger issue of why elderly people exist. Nancy Mergler and Michael Goldstein ask precisely this question.[8] Humans are among the rare species of which a considerable 'post-reproductive cohort' remains alive. This suggests that for a group of humans there may be hidden evolutionary advantages to the presence of older members. If we accept this perspective, then older people must have things to offer that make their presence advantageous. Mergler and Goldstein invite us to see ageing not as deterioration or decline but as a separate phase of development with characteristics of its own. One of those characteristics, they say, is a transition to a more narrative way of passing on information. Another characteristic is the reminiscence effect. Both are said to have adaptive value. It is the task of older people to initiate younger members into the group's social conventions, values and history. Because of the reminiscence effect, they tend to recall precisely those events that are not part of the direct experience of younger people. Seen in this way, the reminiscence effect helps us to pass on knowledge and skills, and to preserve the cohesiveness and identity of the group over time.

It is an explanation that tends in the direction of 'grandpa says'. Older people are believed to enjoy telling stories because children are the best listeners. They like to talk about 'the olden days' because children will hear everything else from their parents. But explanations of this sort should be treated with some scepticism. The dramatic increase in the number of elderly and very elderly people is a relatively recent phenomenon. In evolutionary terms, it was not long ago that having three generations alive at the same time was rare; in fact it is such a recent phenomenon that we cannot credibly make a connection between the characteristics of older people and an evolutionary function.

A purely biological explanation for the origin of the reminiscence bump brings us up against another problem too. If the quality of the memory determines when impressions are most effectively stored, the bump ought to have a different shape. The ripening of the brain, and with it the memory, is appropriately reflected in the left flank of the bump, with an increase in the teenage years, but the slope on the right flank, the descent, does not fit with the decline of the memory, which in reality takes place far more gradually. Most of our memory faculties remain up to scratch for a long time and there is no suggestion that forty-year-olds can store away only a fraction of what they could retain at twenty. There must be other factors at play.

One indication of this comes from experiments involving older people who emigrated after reaching the age of the reminiscence bump. Participants in their mid-sixties who emigrated from Spanish-speaking countries to the United States between the ages of twenty and thirty-five, and had lived in their new country for more than thirty years, were shown a series of cue words intended to release memories.[9] In those who emigrated in their early twenties, the reminiscence bump remained in its usual place: around the age of twenty. Those who left in their mid-thirties showed a different pattern: the bump had shifted to their mid-thirties, at the expense of memories of the time that would in normal circumstances be the reminiscence period. It is highly unlikely that emigration causes a later ripening of the brain, so this outcome is hard to explain based on ideas about the better quality of the young memory. Surely it is more credible to assume that in those who emigrated in their mid-thirties the many new impressions, the new language they had to learn, the social discontinuity, and new circumstances surrounding training, work, housing and daily activities gave them experiences that were stored away even more effectively than those from the time when their memories were at a biological peak. Might not the reminiscence effect therefore have more to do with memorable events than with a receptive brain?

When I was about seventeen I read the memoirs of J.B. Charles about his time in the Dutch wartime resistance.[10] Nowadays I could not tell you much about the content, but one thing that is ingrained on my memory is a passage about how irritating some shy people are. Why are people shy? Because their main concern is what others will think of them. Ultimately they are not interested in those around them, only in what others will conclude about them. If they walk into a room or join a group of people, they are so preoccupied by what these people will think that they start to see themselves from the outside, so to speak, wondering whether they might be blushing or showing other signs of insecurity. Shy people looking at others are looking, through them, at themselves.

After that outburst of irritation from Charles, I could no longer see shyness the way I had always done, as a rather charming quality indicative of sensitivity. It now involved something ambivalent that I indeed found rather unpleasant, even in myself. It made shyness into something other than the opposite of bluntness and insensitivity. There is an aspect to shy people that is less than charming. With this newly acquired insight into the nature of the shy person, something in me changed. Throughout life we find ourselves in situations where we feel shy, but just thinking back to that brief, stinging analysis by Charles works like an index finger wagging admonishingly back and forth in front of my face.

We seem to be more receptive in youth to reading experiences of the kind that change something inside us permanently. The Dutch newspaper *NRC Handelsblad* used to have a series called 'The Decisive Book', in which writers talked about the book that changed their life. 'That whole idea of the decisive book,' said Jessica Durlacher, 'has to do with a decisive time in your life. When are books decisive? Around the age of twenty. You read them differently then, looking for a voice that fits you.'[11] Her own decisive book was *Terug tot Ina Damman* by Simon Vestdijk, which she read at the age of sixteen. Vestdijk creates an atmosphere of menace around the narrator, a boy moving from middle school to high school. It resonated with what Durlacher was feeling at the time. When Arnon Grunberg was fifteen, the first few pages of Henry Miller's *Tropic of Cancer* were enough to make him recognize the author's worldview as his own. At the age of sixteen, Gerrit Krol took 'A Gentle Creature', a story by Dostoyevsky, out of the public library early one Saturday afternoon and finished it about five hours later. He then read it again, reaching the end at about nine in the evening. He recognized himself in the pawnbroker 'who is older and is obeyed by a young girl, although for his part, in bursts of admiration, he sometimes lies at her feet like a floor cloth. I've never done that, but it's in me to want it. Yes, I wanted to be that kind of person'. The difference in age and experience between the character and the reader fell away for Krol: 'I felt: when I get to be that age, I'll be that way too'.[12] Charlotte Mutsaers had forgotten almost everything about *De man die zijn haar kort liet knippen* by Johan Daisne, but she did remember the one curious detail 'that the protagonist, in love, when he is completely coming apart at the seams, seeks treatment at a barber's shop, where his head is massaged with a kind of electric knob'.[13] Daisne's story about a teacher who falls passionately in love with a pupil helped Mutsaers, then fifteen, to interpret her own feelings for her Dutch teacher. 'I'd never spoken to anyone about my own love; I didn't really know what falling in love was about. All I knew was: that must be it, that's what's happened to me, I've fallen in love'.[14] In all the newspaper's conversations about reading, memories like these emerged, featuring passages and characters that changed or clarified the readers' views of themselves.

Of the fifty-one writers, we know the ages of forty-eight when they read their decisive book, and they range from ten to sixty-six. But the tally shows that the decisive books are distributed extremely unevenly over a lifetime; three-quarters of the writers read them before the age of twenty-three and after that age a downward trend quickly sets in. Several were in their thirties, a few in their forties and fifties, and finally there is Hugo Pos, the oldest, who seems to be making a single-handed attempt to refute the reminiscence effect. It would perhaps be going too far to say that by your mid-twenties you are too old to read a decisive book – after all, Cees Nooteboom read Proust at the age of forty – but the median age for 'the book that changed a life' is around nineteen, right at the centre of the reminiscence period.

As part of a Scandinavian study into reading and memory, sixty-six elderly people, with an average age of sixty-eight, were asked to name a book that was connected in their minds with a 'memorable reading experience'.[15] Stretching over seven decades, the ages at which they read those books coincide with the reminiscence curve precisely: less than 5 per cent fall within the first ten years, then there is a sharp increase up into the twenties and thirties, followed by a downward curve, until by about the age of fifty the percentage drops to barely any higher than for children under ten. Right at the end comes the familiar upward sweep of the recency effect. The peak is at

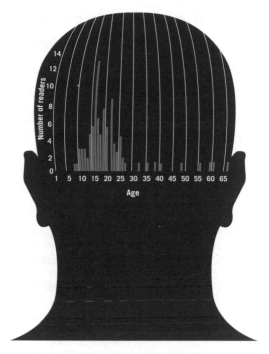

Fig. 3   Age at which interviewees read a 'decisive book'.

thirty, a little later than for the authors interviewed for 'The Decisive Book', but given the literary sensitivity that is a pre-requisite of the writing profession, that may be exactly what one would expect.

There seems to be a sensitive period for pop music just as there is for memorable reading experiences. What people regard as the music of 'my generation' begins at around the time they are fourteen or fifteen and ends in their late twenties, a window of some fifteen years. Their appreciation of that music remains almost constant from then on.[16] If test participants are asked to give their assessment of the quality of hits on a scale ranging from great to abominable, then hits within that window generally tend towards the great and those that come afterwards tend towards the abominable. A graph showing their preferences can be summarized very simply: 'Pop music was at its best when I was around twenty and went downhill rapidly from then on'. Such studies are often derived from market research, since anyone choosing music for use in a commercial aimed at people in their late forties will benefit from the knowledge that 'Sledgehammer' by Peter Gabriel was a hit in 1986. The target group was around twenty then – that ever-shifting cohort lucky enough to have grown up at a time when good music was still being made.

Knowledge of facts about important political or social events follows the same pattern. In an American study, more than a thousand adults were asked to explain in as much detail as possible the significance of the Holocaust, the Marshall Plan, Joe McCarthy, Rosa Parks, the Tet Offensive, My Lai, Woodstock, John Dean and Watergate.[17] The most accurate description was not of the most recent event, which ought to have been freshest in the memory, but of that which happened when the participant was in his or her mid-twenties. The vortex effect of events from that time was so powerful that even mistakes in dating them seemed to be the result of age. Quite a few people who were in their mid-twenties in the mid-1950s placed the Tet Offensive during the Korean War (1950–53). In reality, of course, it took place in 1968, during the Vietnam War.

This formation of literary and musical preferences and shared memories of political or social events creates something that each of us could call 'my era'. Almost a hundred people aged between twenty-six and sixty-seven were asked to put together a list of five films they regarded as typical of 'their era'.[18] They were instructed to choose films they would recommend others to go and see in order to gain a better understanding of what inspired them and their contemporaries. The question of what exactly was meant by 'their era' was deliberately left vague. For practically everyone, 'my era' turned out to coincide with the years of the reminiscence bump. On average the respondents were twenty when the film of 'their era' came out.

People in a position to talk about a long career locate events they regard as having had important consequences for them in the period when their careers had barely taken off. An analysis of forty-nine autobiographical texts written by eminent psychologists has shown that they often had 'flashbulb memories' of such events.[19] These were usually experiences from their student years, which for most of them meant some fifty years ago. As with the decisive book, there seems to be a time for what will later be remembered as the decisive meeting, the pivotal event, the crucial conversation that made apparent something about yourself, your life or your plans. That time is when you were in your early twenties.

In autobiographies, memoirs and interviews, such recollections are easy to single out; they could even be categorized by type and subtype. There are hurtful experiences recalled in order to explain a persistent aversion to someone or something, as distinct from hurtful experiences dredged up with feelings of triumph. Basketball player Michael Jordan has described how he failed the selection for the college team in his second year: 'They posted the roster and it was there for a long, long time without my name on it. I remember being really mad, too, because there was a guy who made it that really wasn't as good as me. . . . Whenever I was working out and got tired and figured I ought to stop, I'd close my eyes and see that list in the locker room without my name on it, and that usually got me going again.'[20] Another regular feature of the autobiographical genre is the memory of 'where it all started', such as a meeting that made someone decide to study medicine, become a mechanic or train as a musician. Other events enter the memory – and often the autobiography or the story people tell about themselves – as 'life lessons'. These are things you picked up, usually at a young age, that continued to guide you when you were faced with a choice. The 'turning point' is another element that features in almost every life story: the conversation that made you switch subjects at university, the incident that persuaded you to leave your job, the exchange of words that put an end to a friendship. But what all these experiences have in common, no matter how diverse and no matter whether they are spoken of, written about or kept secret, is that they occur most frequently in the years covered by the reminiscence bump.

Psychologists Dorthe Berntsen and David Rubin have made a bold attempt to play off the different interpretations of the reminiscence bump against one another.[21] If the neurological receptivity of a young brain is sufficient by itself to explain the reminiscence effect, then you would expect the nature of the memories themselves to make little difference. Whether happy or sad, traumatic or important, they would be easy to recall later because they became stuck in the mind at the right moment. Events that were perhaps just as intense but experienced twenty years later would slip loose from the memory, leaving barely a trace. As the shifting of the reminiscence bump by emigration has already suggested, this explanation raises quite a few questions, and Berntsen and Rubin have their doubts too. They interviewed 1,241 Danes aged between twenty and ninety-three and asked them to think about their saddest, happiest and most important memories, and to say how old they were at the time. Contrary to what we would predict based on the biological explanation, the spread of those memories across a lifetime was quite diverse.

The happiest memory followed the pattern of the reminiscence bump even in people still in their thirties. After a peak at around the age of twenty-five, the curve began to turn downwards again. The older the age group, the more clearly defined the reminiscence bump. The peak lay in the mid-twenties and it did not shift, instead becoming increasingly prominent as the decades went by. Memories of the most important event produced a similar curve, with a peak at around the age of twenty-five, once again highest for the older age groups. But the curve for the saddest memory followed a different pattern. It rose uniformly for every age group, which means that the chance of a memory being regarded as 'the saddest memory' increased to the degree that the event had occurred recently.

This pattern was found in earlier research too. In an experiment in which a hundred people aged between fifty-five and seventy-eight were asked to identify their best and worst memories, the most pleasant memory followed the pattern of the reminiscence curve, whereas the curve for the worst memory flattened out after they turned twenty. In the study already mentioned, in which people were required to name four memories they would definitely want to include in their autobiography, it turned out that in three-quarters of cases the memory was distinctly pleasant. The explanation for this cannot simply be that more unpleasant things happen to you as you get older, since the effect was the same for every age group and it is unlikely, Berntsen and Rubin write, that over the previous ten or twenty years, life in Denmark had taken a turn for the worse for all of them. The researchers checked to be sure, and confirmed that it was an era of declining unemployment, increasing prosperity and a falling suicide rate.

So where does this odd discrepancy come from? Why do people locate their best, happiest and most important memories in their youth and their saddest memories so much closer to the present day? Berntsen and Rubin can do little more than establish that the difference exists. Is it because we tend to share our happiest memories with others and therefore remember them better? Do we prefer not to talk or think too much about the most unhappy moments in our lives? Do we have a worse memory for unpleasant events? Do sad times have different or even perhaps no consequences at all for the 'story of your life'? Whatever the explanation, the curve for the saddest of memories is difficult to reconcile with a biological theory about the brain that shows little distinction between the three types and regards the memory as most effective at around the age of twenty and starting to lose strength after that.

Despite all this, the neurological receptiveness of a young brain is not irrelevant to the reminiscence effect. Whatever it is that gives a book, a meeting or an incident its decisive character is not dependent on neurological factors, but the fact that once such things have been experienced as decisive they are then stored away more effectively may indeed be the result of receptivity in the brain. The same applies to memories of 'first times'. Naturally there are more 'first times' when you are twenty than when you are fifty, but they are also better recorded in the memory at around that age, which almost amounts to a guarantee that memories of 'first times' will later, when we look back, make a significant contribution to the reminiscence bump.

If we accept this explanation – that memorable events and experiences which in themselves have nothing to do with neurological ripening are nevertheless reinforced by it – then the question arises as to whether the reminiscence effect might not be noticeable even in someone of thirty or forty. Controversy is currently raging over this very point. One line of research suggests that 'young' memories are over-represented from the moment they come into being.[22] Initially they are not visible as that neat 'bump' of thirty or forty years later, simply because they still coincide with the upward sweep of the recency effect. Another line of research indicates that only towards the age of sixty do early memories start to be over-represented, coming to mind with the realization 'I haven't thought about that for fifty years'. Neither set of studies has presented a decisive outcome as yet. The reminiscence effect may be as old as humanity, but research into it is still young.

The question of exactly when the reminiscence effect comes into play has yet to be settled among psychologists, but because our populations are ageing, we now know more about how the effect progresses once it has started. The rapid increase in the number of very elderly people is presenting psychology with new experimental opportunities. In the West at least, we now have a cohort of people with extremely old memories, and this offers us the chance to examine whether the reminiscence effect continues to increase as we become very elderly, or levels off. As far back as 1967, two American researchers managed to find more than 276 centenarians willing to take part in an experiment.[23] They asked these participants to recall the most exciting event in their lives. The period up to the age of forty turned out to contain 70 per cent of such memories and the sixty years that followed only 30 per cent.

In 2003 several Danish centenarians were questioned about their memories.[24] Their answers were compared to those given by a group of eighty-year-olds. Both groups clearly demonstrated the reminiscence effect, but in the centenarians that effect was even stronger than among the 'youngsters' of eighty (see Figure 2).

The Danish researchers also discovered an intriguing illustration of the power of the reminiscence effect. Asked about important public events in their lifetimes, around half of the eighty-year-olds talked about memories that had to do with the German occupation during the Second World War. None of the centenarians did so. In a different experimental setting, words such as 'flag' and 'money' elicited just one memory of the Second World War among the hundred-year-olds but four of the unification of Jutland with Denmark in 1920, which happened when they were around twenty. Bearing the reminiscence effect in mind, it is easy to imagine what is going on here. For those aged eighty, the war fell neatly within the reminiscence bump. The centenarians were already in their forties by then. It is age, rather than the gravity of the circumstances, that seems to be the most important factor when it comes to what we remember best in old age.

The reporting of memories in any detail is actually quite rare in psychological literature about the reminiscence effect. As a rule they are all tallied up and laid out in histograms that show the distribution of memories over the decades of a lifetime. Anyone wanting to read about the content of those reminiscences would do better to consult the interviews collected by Steffie van den Oord in her book *Eeuwelingen* (*Centenarians*).[25] She spoke to twenty-two people aged a hundred or more. The oldest, Hendrikje Schipper, was born in 1890 and others were born in 1891, 1893 and 1896. The things they talked about issued from extremely old memories, so they are a window on a world that hardly anyone else knows first-hand. Hendrikje Schipper remembered a farmer who ordered a bicycle from the Fongers bicycle factory and took the barge to Groningen every day for a week, where he was taught to cycle. She herself bought a vacuum cleaner in 1926, a Hoover, and went to the vacuum cleaning school for two days to learn to use it: 'Don't push it quickly back and forth but move the machine gently across the floor, otherwise the dust doesn't have time to get inside.'[26]

Many of the memories are recounted with the open-heartedness of old age. Pieter Schoonewille from Noordscheschut in Drenthe, born in 1901, carried the milk churns from sixty small farmers to the steam-powered cooperative dairy plant Erica 2 on his barge, four hours there, four hours back, six days a week. Schoonewille, father of five children, told Van den Oord that he had never yet seen a naked woman in the flesh. 'I've slept with my wife often enough, but I've never, ever seen her naked. That might seem ridiculous to you now, but it wasn't then. We took baths separately too, in a half-barrel. Why? Embarrassment perhaps. I don't really know. But I don't regret it in the least. Later I did sometimes see naked women of course; nowadays you commonly see them on television.'[27] When Schoonewille became a widower at the age of seventy, he found himself a new girlfriend, but it came to nothing: the old milk-churn bargee soon realized she was only in it for the sex.

Anyone using these interviews as a source of knowledge about the workings of memory at an advanced age has to take into account all kinds of possible bias. Some stories may reflect the interests of the interviewer rather than the people she interviewed. Perhaps the centenarians were put firmly into reverse gear by opening questions such as 'What is your earliest memory?' Since one memory leads to another, much of what followed from that first memory would also be from early childhood. With centenarians this is probably more the case than usual, simply because the sensational thing about their memories is precisely that they go so far back. But even with these reservations in mind, we can find many things in these conversations that have wider application for psychologists looking at elderly memories.

In these interviewees, who were elderly even in 1960, the reminiscence effect assumes almost hilarious proportions. Louis Hellebrekers, a brickmaker born in 1901, says that the hot summer of 1911 is still fresh in his mind: 'It was so terribly dry – you could toss your hat and it'd catch on the cow's hip'.[28] His right arm is starting to weaken, incidentally: he worked it too hard in 1916. Jan Pieter Bos, born in 1891, who was a bargeman on the inland waterways, can describe in detail the wooden sailing boat his father captained, but not how old he was when he finally got married: 'Not till I was thirty-nine, I think'.[29] Sophie Smit can still remember moving out of the town of Zierikzee, but she has forgotten all about moving back after retiring from her office job, fifty years closer to the present day.

When these centenarians talk about 'the war' they mean not the Second World War but the First, when Dutch military activities were limited to mobilization. It is ingrained on their memories. At the age of thirteen, Louis Hellebrekers stood at a station in Germany watching young men leave for the trenches in France, and in his dreams he still sometimes sees the weeping women and children left behind on the platform. Other centenarians tell stories about Belgian refugees, food distribution and rationing, the minefields at Dogger Bank, the shortage of coal, or the conscription that interrupted their higher education or apprenticeships. For cheesemaker Annigje Baron-Rozendaal (born in 1893) trade came to a standstill; she spent four years doing embroidery. Most are noticeably less voluble about the Second World War, when they were in their forties and fifties. Some seem to recall little more about that war than that it started in May 1940 (when the Germans invaded the Netherlands), and ended five years later.

The reminiscence effect can be seen in every one of these interviews and it is sometimes very prominent. Van den Oord talked to Cornelia van het Westeinde-Vermue, a robust woman from the province of Zeeland, born in Kruiningen in 1899. She has brought up ten children and still wears traditional dress. She talks nineteen to the dozen until the subject of the great flooding disaster comes up. Cornelia is startled: 'The flood?'[30] She turns pale. Her voice shaking, she describes how bigger and bigger waves came over the dyke, the polder filled with water and she ran home as quickly as she could. When it got dark, the children climbed into bed together, listening to their father, who walked back and forth along the top of the dyke all night. She starts to cry and stops speaking. Her daughter, in her eighties herself, is listening in: 'Mother tells this story every week and even now she can't help crying'.[31] It all seems perfectly understandable to the Dutch reader, except that later in the story it turns out that she is not talking about the famous flood of 1953, but about a dyke that burst in 1906. One polder flooded and a few chickens drowned, whereas the 1953 disaster killed 1,800 people. When Van den Oord asks about that event, Cornelia says: 'No, I don't remember the 1953 flood as well as the 1906 flood. It was such a storm that the dyke swayed back and forth! Really, it did'.[32] It seems as if the crystal-clear visibility of 1906 demands the relative invisibility of 1953, as if the remembering of one event requires the forgetting of the other.

Take the story of Douwe van der Wielen, who was able to claim he had lived in three centuries. He was born fifteen minutes before the turn of the twentieth century in the village of Bergum in Friesland and died on 3 January 2001. As a fifteen-year-old he heard a new church minister's inaugural sermon and from that moment on he wanted to be a pastor. He tells a moving story about the efforts made by his father and brothers to enable him to study, how his brother Jochem at first escaped the mobilization by drawing lot number 84 ('Tietjerksteradeel was required to provide eighty-three recruits') but then had to report for duty after all because someone had died. He still remembers the precise timetable of the regular barge service his father ran, and what tea cost per ounce and coffee per half pound. Then his story reaches the year 1944. By that time he was a pastor in Boornbergum. The suspension of a particular theology professor threatened to cause a schism in his parish, as it had elsewhere. There is no doubt that at the time Reverend Van der Wielen knew exactly what the conflict was all about, but he has forgotten now: 'To be honest, I don't know any longer exactly what the difference of opinion was. Your memory does after all take a knock.'[33] Indeed, it is hard to decide which is the more astonishing: the persistence of his oldest memories or the lacunase, bordering on amnesia, when he talks about the period of his middle age.

The explanation given by Cornelia, from Zeeland, still weeping about a dyke that broke when she was seven, is disarmingly simple. She puts her hand to her heart: 'In 1906 I still had room here to remember everything.'[34] It is a notion that echoes the biological explanation of the reminiscence effect: the young memory is still capable of storing things away in great detail. But the stories told by centenarians also lend support to other, rather more intricate explanations. One thing that strikes the reader, for example, is the frequency of memories of 'first times'. Almost everyone can recall their first day at school, their first meeting with the man or woman they would later marry, their first day in a new job. Sea captain Tigchelaar (born in 1897) describes winning his first sextant in an exam at nautical college. Bicycle-maker Nijk from Steggerda (born in 1900) still remembers the licence plate of his first car, in 1926 – B 12470 – but not those of any of his subsequent vehicles. Sister Fintana (born in 1900) recalls seeing nuns for the first time in 1908. Reverend Van der Wielen says that he first saw electric light at a travelling cinema. You can point to this phenomenon in all the interviews. Hendrikje Schipper remembers her first tomatoes and how her mother threw away the first crop of the unnerving fruit: 'I'm not eating that stuff; they're just like oranges.'[35] Van der Goes van Naters, the 'red nobleman', born in 1900, vividly remembers the first worker he ever met.

No less striking is that memories of insults and affronts, which the centenarians describe in detail with little prompting, almost always relate to events from the reminiscence period. Sophie Smit had a teacher ('Miss Krensen, I'll never forget her') who promised her a present. When it finally came it was a gnawed stump of pencil: 'Rubbish! When I got home I threw it away in the corner.'[36] Antoon Brunia, born in 1900, served in the hussars as a young farrier. He starts telling an elaborate story about his disputes with a captain of horse – 'one of those upper-class types' – who tried to have him demoted to blacksmith's assistant. He becomes so involved in his story that he finds himself able to quote their altercations at length ('I still get mad as I tell it'). How reliable all those memories are is a different matter, but they undoubtedly feel vivid and real. What the centenarians, looking back, see as the greatest affronts to them were experienced early in life.

There is a third category too, a prominent feature of these particular reminiscences, namely events that gave a life a decisive change of tack. For Van der Goes van Naters it was a fiery speech by Pieter Jelles Troelstra in Nijmegen, which marked the start of a long career in Socialist politics. For Sophie Smit it was her first job interview at a mortgage bank; for bicycle-maker Nijk his father's decision that he, just turned fourteen, would have to come and work at the factory, since his two older brothers had been called up. Sister Fintana remembers vividly the moment when, at the age of twenty-one, after summoning courage for seven years, she told her mother she wanted to enter a convent. The first meeting with a future husband or wife, a conversation that has a huge and lasting influence on your political beliefs – many reminiscences concern events that tend to happen more often in childhood and early adulthood than later, and are generally not repeated.

None of these centenarians has written an autobiography, yet the stories of their lives have the usual cast of characters and twists and turns that we see in the autobiographical genre. The event that started it all, the turning point, the moment that brought about a complete change of course, the meeting that was to have important consequences, the lesson for life, even the insults that seem to make so much more of an impression in youth – they emerge of their own accord when the centenarians look back over their long lives. And even in these unwritten autobiographies they take their traditional place: the opening chapters.

Reminiscences are a triple enigma. They come back at a time when other memory skills are declining. They are not the product of deterioration in once intact faculties but truly new and therefore, mercifully, they put the notion of a parabolic pattern into perspective; and, no less puzzlingly, it is precisely those early memories that seem successfully to resist forgetting. Most remarkable of all perhaps is the realization that as the reminiscence effect attains its full force, memories will return to which you have long been denied access. These are memories that really do slumber. They were laid down in every detail, but kept under embargo. People aged forty or fifty may think they are standing on the top step of the staircase of life and experiencing events of great weight and moment, but twenty years later, when the sealed envelopes are opened, it turns out that they think back mainly to what they went through as teenagers and young adults. That the average person rarely takes much account of this is a blessing in disguise. You might not want to be operated on by a surgeon aged forty who is thinking: 'Well, what does it matter? I'll have forgotten all about this in thirty years from now.'

Anyone who looks at the curve representing the memories of the Danish centenarians will notice a rather dispiriting detail at the bottom right. What hundred-year-olds have gained compared to eighty-year-olds is another twenty years that produce few memories. In calendar terms those are the same twenty years as between birth and the age of twenty, but to the memory the first twenty are an eternity, the last twenty a mere sigh. Van den Oord found the same phenomenon in her centenarians. They are of course a little surprised at how much they have forgotten about the second half of their lives, despite the fact that those years included dramatic events such as the great flood or the German occupation. In the case of Annigje, the cheesemaker, the memories that are worth talking about seem to stop in the 1930s: 'After that not very much else happened. I lived outside Rotterdam during the Second World War, safe with my family. I can't remember much about it. I don't recall everything about the war by any means. The first man on the moon? I wouldn't know any longer. I haven't kept track of everything. Why would I?'[37] Bear in mind that this is her summary of a full sixty years.

With all that forgetting, many centenarians have the impression that their extremely long lives have flown by. As if to confirm that life speeds up as we get older, one of them says: 'It may sound ridiculous, but I can't fathom how short life is, really, even though mine has lasted more than a hundred years.'[38]

CHAPTER FIVE

The joy of calling up memories

Elderly people, wrote Aristotle, 'live by memory rather than by hope; for what is left to them of life is but little as compared with the long past; and hope is of the future, memory of the past. This, again, is the cause of their loquacity; they are continually talking of the past, because they enjoy remembering it'.[1] The quotation comes from his *Rhetoric*: good rhetoricians must have a feeling for what is going on in their listeners' heads, whether or not they happen to be old. Anyone turning to this passage in the hope of finding something more encouraging about old people would do well to skip the section about 'The character of Elderly Men', as it only gets worse. The elderly are distrustful, since they have frequently been taken in and know that 'life on the whole is a bad business'. They are greedy, because they know from experience how hard it is to acquire money and how easy to lose it. If they give the impression that they lead lives of moderation and self-control, then it is only because 'their passions have slackened'. They have sympathy with their fellow man, but only because they are always aware that what happens to others could easily happen to them. Above all, they talk a lot about the past.

Of course a good rhetorician also needs to know the characteristics of young people, and they turn out to be just as unpleasant as those of the elderly. Young people are hot-tempered, with a tendency to succumb to their anger. They love honour and cannot bear being slighted. Since there are few occasions on which they have been cheated, they are too trusting of others. They have powerful desires and give in to them too readily. Their attitude to memory is the reverse of that of elderly people: 'Their lives are mainly spent not in memory but in expectation; for expectation refers to the future, memory to the past, and youth has a long future before it and a short past behind it: on the first day of one's life one has nothing at all to remember, and can only look forward.'[2]

Halfway between the first light of day and the evening of life lies middle age, which Aristotle calls our 'prime'. The character of a man in the prime of life is just right. He is neither too trusting nor too distrustful, neither rash nor timid, given neither to parsimony nor to prodigality. The characteristics of youth and old age are in a happy balance and appropriately combined. 'The body is in its prime from thirty to five-and-thirty; the mind about forty-nine.'[3] Aristotle is believed to have written this part of his *Rhetoric* when he was aged around forty, just past his physical prime, with his mental prime still to come. He was, in everything, a man of the golden mean.

In a series of journal entries by the Swiss writer Max Frisch in which he writes, in the style of a novel, about a hypothetical Voluntary Death Society, the protagonist makes a discovery. Once into his sixties he sees that characteristics he has tended to attribute to a person's nature – someone is ambitious, generous or unflappable – are actually a matter of age. He notices this in himself as well. When he compares his current self with his earlier self, he realizes that there are aspects to his personality that have appeared and disappeared. It seems these were not part of his character. He has been 'mistaking age-related personality traits for personal characteristics'.[4] This is the essence of what Aristotle meant. A person is not gullible or greedy by nature but rather by age.

Other passages likewise make it seem as if Frisch is writing a novel based on Aristotle's *Rhetoric*. Young and old have different relationships with past and future. For a young person, Frisch writes, the future is 'a sum total of vague possibilities (at a certain point he'll get married, it might be later, or perhaps never, perhaps he'll become famous, perhaps not, perhaps he'll emigrate somewhere or other)'. For an older person the future is 'everything for which he is no longer eligible, the sum total of definite impossibilities (he'll never learn to fly a glider, he'll never see a man land on Mars, nor even the new Zurich Central Station, and so on)'.[5]

Anyone who decides not to read about this hypothetical society because of its rather grim title will be missing out. Frisch gives voice to the experience of growing older in such a witty and playful way that even those of us who are well past the age when we are likely to read our decisive book will find insights here that cause a shift in our thinking about old age. Frisch turned sixty in 1971 and was drawing upon his own personal experience.

The Voluntary Death Society is a club that the protagonist has set up to combat the ageing of the population. Now that medical science allows us to become older than anyone would want to be, members are expected to take responsibility when the time comes to do their bit to make society younger. It has fallen to the narrator, the only writer among them, to put together a handbook for members and aspiring members, and to draw up the statutes. This is no easy task. How old is old? How old is too old?

Anyone aged over fifty can join the club. Members meet twice a year 'to draw each other's attention to signs of old age in them'.[6] If one of their number keeps prolonging his life, they cannot demand that he end it voluntarily, but the annual meeting may decide that he has violated the statutes. This requires a two-thirds majority in a secret ballot. If the member persists he will be expelled from the club. The member can appeal, and the appeals process includes an additional test: a speech 'on a subject of his own choosing, that will not be judged on the basis of oratorical skill, often seen in the elderly, but on an ability or inability to see an issue differently from the day before, and to cast doubt upon his own answers of the previous day. . . . If in his speech there is not even the hint of a new thought that he previously regarded as unthinkable, he will be considered an old man'.[7] All members take a written test to determine whether or not they can express themselves in the language current at that moment. Lists will have to be compiled of outdated terms, which it is predicted will eventually include 'learning process' and 'polarize', for example. The decline of members' mental faculties is measured at every meeting by a memory test. As early as the very first annual meeting, the procedures have to be adjusted. The speech is scrapped. 'An unexpected phenomenon: quick-wittedness in the elderly. Anyone aged over sixty has learned to answer questions with appropriate answers to questions that were not asked; this creates an impression of mental activity.'[8]

In the handbook and the statutes, and indeed in the narrator's remarks, the problems used to define 'too old' are, invariably, memory problems. Not being able to remember names is an ominous sign. 'Hardly anyone who takes the floor as a full member can speak for fifteen minutes without having to ask: What's that place called again? . . . Then, over dinner: His name eludes me, but you know who I mean, so that's all right. And ten minutes later, when the conversation has moved on, it comes to him: Jünger's his name, Ernst Jünger, not the other one, that's his brother. It's all quite laborious.'[9] The members have more success at pretending to have good memories. They like to talk, drawing on a large repertoire of anecdotes, mostly concerning events of long ago. These are not really memories but something resembling memories of memories, so the members repeat them-selves, word for word. A decision is made to tape-record the evening meetings: 'a note will be made of anyone who recounts the same youthful memory more than three times.'[10]

With his observations on memory and old age, Max Frisch almost effortlessly closes the gap of twenty-three centuries since Aristotle warned about loquacious elderly people who enjoy recounting past experiences.

Three years before Frisch started writing journal entries about his approaching old age, Aristotle's name appeared in an article by American psychiatrist Robert Butler about elderly people and reminiscences.[11] In the still-young geriatric tradition to which Butler belonged, reminiscences were seen as part of a tendency among older people to look back and take stock of their lives, usually referred to as a 'life review'. The word 'review' has a dual meaning: a re-examination but also a definitive verdict. Butler believed that the former was in the service of the latter. He certainly did not regard this tendency to look back as having exclusively beneficial effects. In his opening paragraph he refers to Aristotle's explanation: the short future and the long past. In residential homes it seems to be young staff members and young therapists who find it particularly difficult to listen to the residents' long stories.

Interpreted negatively like this, there is something involun-tary about reminiscence. It happens to an elderly person sponta-neously and indiscriminately, which suggests it is an unconscious mechanism that allows older people to escape for a while from some of the more unpleasant aspects of their current lives. Butler thought of reminiscence as a return to past events and experiences, and above all to unresolved conflicts that could now at last be put right, although this brought with it a danger that the older people concerned would reach too negative a verdict on their lives. In severe cases depression might result. Butler made a connection with fear of death. The end is now very close and that in itself, in some sense, forces a person to look back. The conclusion drawn would depend on what the individual concerned 'saw' in his or her past life. Looking back might lead to sadness, remorse, regret or despair, but happier outcomes were possible: satisfaction, a sense of fulfilment, closure. Sometimes a sharper image would be created of the ambitions and aspirations of earlier years, and with it an ability to determine what came of them and why things did not turn out as planned.

Until the late 1960s, there was a strong tendency to discourage reminiscence, since it was seen as diverting elderly people from the immediate demands of the present day, and even of speeding the deterioration of cognitive processes that are much needed in later life.[12] It was also said to present an unpleasant contrast to current circumstances. The discovery that the move from independent living to a care home has a deleterious effect on short-term memory and concentration, and that after the move there is a tendency for an elderly person to become increasingly lost in memories, seemed to underline the danger of reminiscence. In short, the verdict of geriatricians and psychiatrists on thinking and talking about the old days was hardly any more positive than Aristotle's.

The tide turned in the 1980s and 1990s. From many sides simultaneously, and often on the initiative of therapists working in residential homes for elderly people, the recalling of early memories began to be encouraged. Sometimes old people were invited to tell their life stories or write them down. Guidebooks appeared that explained how to lead such projects; in fact many countries now have publishing houses that specialize in the life stories of elderly people, mostly in limited print-runs for family and friends. Photographs, old film footage or music may help to unlock memories. Many old people's homes now have memory cabinets or special rooms with old tools and utensils that were once found in every household but disappeared half a century ago, bottles containing smells of the past, washing powders with once popular brand names, sounds that long ago disappeared from our streets, or photographs of people who were famous in the 1920s and 1930s. Words or terms that refer to things that no longer exist and therefore have meaning only in the memory are used to get conversations going in 'reminiscence groups'. One generation still knows them, the next no longer does. Examples might include platform ticket, winding wool, Player's Navy Cut, ash bucket and meat safe.

Sometimes memories are the only means left of reaching an elderly person. In those with mild dementia, very early recollections are often still accessible, so efforts can be made to deploy them for therapeutic purposes. One example in the Netherlands is the project 'Geheugen in Beeld' ('Memory in Pictures'), set up by a nursing home in cooperation with the Archive of the Province of Drenthe, which has digitized a large proportion of its photographic collection. Its website (www.drentsarchief.nl) enables staff to look for photographs from the precise region, village or town where an old person grew up. This approach, involving group conversations prompted by historical photographs, has an astonishingly stimulating effect on elderly people in the early stages of dementia – as I was able to see for myself when I was invited to join one such session.

The women – there was only one man in the group – introduced themselves by their full names. They had forenames typical of the region: Aaltje, Berendina, Jantje. Only a few used the surnames that had been theirs throughout marriage, those of their late husbands. Mrs Dantuma-Schipper is Aaltje Schipper again after fifty or sixty years, as if there never was a Mr Dantuma. The therapists had prepared me for the fact that the women had reverted to their childhoods. They were more likely to talk about their parents than about their children, more likely to describe their brothers and sisters in childhood than to make any reference to their own grandchildren. They had returned to primary-school age, as it were, so even asking them how they met their husbands would usually prompt little in the way of recollection.

When the photographs are laid on the table, their faces become expressive again. They lean forward, curious. The first

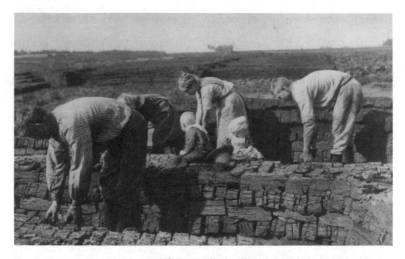

Fig. 4 Peat-cutters in Valthermond, the Netherlands, 1910–20.

photograph, which shows a family piling up slabs of peat, immediately causes a stir. Some of them worked as peat-cutters themselves, or used peat as fuel to heat their homes. Tools like the 'peat iron' come up in the conversation, or *'bollejagen'*, a reference to the noisy protests used to call peat cutters out on strike. Both terms fell into disuse at least two generations ago. They like to explain things to the therapists, especially the older ones who themselves grew up with sacks of coke pellets. For one of the women the photo revives memories of heavy, physically demanding work. As well as cutting peat she was made to help dig potatoes. During her schooldays there was still a 'potato-lifting holiday': 'hard times'. She does not like thinking back to those days. A second photo-graph, of a potato-flour factory called Hollandia in Nieuw-Buinen, is recognized by almost everybody. The one man present turns out to have lived in the factory's tied cottage. He was 'Hollandia's sales manager' and can still describe precisely how he walked into the factory from his house without having to go outdoors. When he is asked whether he was forced to move out of the house when he retired, he becomes confused. He can't recollect that time very well.

After looking at just two photographs it is almost impossible to believe that these are the same people who were sitting in the recreation room silent and apathetic just a quarter of an hour ago. They talk about their childhoods, exchange details about where they grew up, discover that they lived close to each other or went to the same school, perhaps even had the same teacher. Almost all of them can still remember their address, or rather their parents' address. The beginnings of dementia and the historical photographs have combined to transport them back to the 1920s. Their stories feature long-forgotten shop names, places where they go shopping in their memories. The humiliations they remember, great or small, have to do with class or gender distinctions: not being allowed to sit in certain pews in church, having to eat in the kitchen, being forced to leave school because they were girls. But even their unpleasant memories are eagerly recalled and exchanged.

In the guidebook that accompanies the project, psychogeriatrician Henk Loning writes that an elderly person in a care home is forced to operate within dependent relationships. In conversations about old photographs, that dependency falls away. 'Elderly people with dementia are experts on the photograph, which provides a link with their earlier life and their current perception of the world. They inform others about the memories that the photograph automatically draws to the surface. This change in social role confers self-confidence, supports a sense of self-esteem and stimulates feelings of connection and security.'[13]

To be honest, the beneficial effects are fleeting. People with dementia not only have little future (despite perhaps being quite some years away from death), they have a shorter and shorter past as well. The photographs briefly take them back in time and sometimes their memories are so vivid that it seems as if the past has entered the present. But that present is narrow, it can retain little, and soon even the oldest memories will be gone. Only then will all the talk about the old days that so irritated Aristotle finally cease.

CHAPTER SIX

The good son:
A conversation with Oliver Sacks

Anyone starting to write an autobiography will see memories as the raw material available to work on. But the motive for writing an autobiography often seems to arise from the precise opposite: memories that work on the writer.

'In 1993, approaching my sixtieth birthday', wrote Oliver Sacks, looking back on the writing of his autobiography *Uncle Tungsten*, 'I started to experience a curious phenomenon – the spontaneous, unsolicited rising of early memories into my mind, memories which had lain dormant for upwards of fifty years. Not merely memories, but frames of mind, thoughts, atmospheres, and passions associated with them – memories, especially, of my boyhood.'[1] Giving in to his impulse, first with a few short, partly autobiographical passages about the places and people of his childhood, between 1997 and 2000 Sacks chronicled the first fifteen years of his life. Not until the age of eighteen did he start to write letters and keep notebooks, so he had to reconstruct his boyhood years from memories that in many cases could not be checked against documentation. He knew he would have forgotten a great deal, and that his memories would have become less reliable over time, but Sacks is a sensitive observer, even when it comes to the behaviour of his own memory. He takes account of the fact that many memories do not return to our consciousness in a pure, unadulterated form. As a boy of twelve he was already aware of the transformations that objects, people and places can undergo in our memories – it was his most important reason for taking up photography. On the morning of his twelfth birthday, he writes in *Uncle Tungsten*, he took photographs from his bedroom window in Mapesbury Road in north-west London. 'I wished to document, to hold forever, exactly what confronted me when I opened the curtains that morning. (I still have this photo, two photos, actually, designed to form a stereo pair, as a red and a green anaglyph. Now, more than half a century later, it has almost replaced the actual memory, so that if I close my eyes and try to visualize the Mapesbury Road of my boyhood, all I see is the photograph I took.)'[2]

Oliver Sacks was born in London in 1933. His father was a general practitioner, his mother a surgeon. He was part of a large Jewish family on his mother's side. His uncles were chemists, inventors and academics, his aunts doctors and founders of schools. In *Uncle Tungsten*, named after Uncle Dave who owned a factory that made tungsten lamps, Sacks writes that he grew up with a sense that it was some kind of family duty to be 'scientific'.[3]

The Second World War marked the end of what had until then been a happy childhood. His parents sent him and his brother Michael to a boarding school called Braefield in the English Midlands, where they hoped their sons would be safe from the Blitz. Oliver, who would have preferred to be in danger with his parents than safe without them, felt exiled and spent four miserable years at a school where he was bullied by fellow pupils and by a sadistic headmaster.

The end of the war was the start of what Sacks calls his 'chemical boyhood'. He was enthralled by the periodic table. It gave him a sense of order and predictability in a world that had proved to be unstable and dangerous. Young Oliver regularly visited the Science Museum in South Kensington, where one display cabinet covered the entire wall above the stairs. It contained ninety elements laid out according to the system devised by Mendeleev. In his home laboratory he experimented with the most diverse chemicals, initially taking no precautions at all other than to keep the door to the garden open. After one experiment went spectacularly wrong, he was given a fume cupboard and the advice to use rather smaller quantities in future.

Uncle Tungsten comes to an end at the point when Oliver reaches puberty. His passion for chemistry ended fairly abruptly then too. After secondary school he studied medicine at Oxford before leaving for America in the early 1960s. In 1965 he became an instructor at the Albert Einstein College of Medicine in the

Bronx, New York, while at the same time working as a consultant at the Little Sisters of the Poor and at the Beth Abraham Hospital, also in the Bronx. It was at the Beth Abraham that he carried out the experiments with L-dopa that led to his book *Awakenings* (1973), later filmed with Robin Williams in the role of Dr Malcolm Sayer, who was based on Sacks. He decided early on to become an author of books rather than a co-author of articles. *The Man Who Mistook his Wife for a Hat* marked his break-through to a wide readership in 1985. It was only then that Sacks, at the age of fifty-two, was appointed professor of neurology.

In the summer of 2007, Sacks left the Albert Einstein College after a career that had lasted for forty-two years. Not to retire – for the son of a surgeon who was still performing operations at the age of seventy-five and a doctor who practised until he turned ninety that was not the next logical step – but to take up a new post at Columbia University, specially created for him, in which he acts as an intermediary between neuroscience and art. In his lectures he drew upon *Musicophilia*, his tenth book, about the brain and music. Since then Sacks has written two further books: *The Mind's Eye* and *Hallucinations*. He is also still active as a professor at the NYU School of Medicine and as a consulting neurologist at the NYU Langone Medical Center.

It is difficult to name a subject in the field of neurology that Sacks has not explored: migraine, the syndromes named after Tourette, Asperger and Korsakov, Alzheimer's disease, Parkinson's disease, autism, the savant syndrome, phantom pain, colour blindness. His method, which has long fallen into disuse elsewhere, is that of the house call. Sacks travels to visit his patients and spends time with them in their own environments. He has observed operations performed by a surgeon with Tourette's, watched the autistic cattle expert Temple Grandin at work designing cowsheds, visited an island with a large community of totally colour-blind people, travelled to Moscow with an autistic savant artist. He watches, listens, talks and then records his findings in case studies that do justice to both the sickness and the sick. By making house calls, it turns out, Oliver Sacks is following in his father's footsteps.

When Oliver Sacks came to the University of Groningen in October 2005 to give a talk, he agreed to meet me for a conversation about what time does to memories and what memories do to time. It was an unexpectedly sombre affair. Sacks felt ill, which seemed to reinforce his tendency to contemplate his relationship with his parents, the course his life has taken, and old age. His regular travelling companion and editor Kate Edgar wrote later that she had found his mood during our conversation 'uncharacteristically melancholy'.

In a life on the road, Sacks tries to hold on to a couple of habits from home. He does not like to interrupt his psychoanalysis, so when travelling he phones his therapist in New York twice a week. The other habit is his daily swim, which lasts an hour. Each morning of his visit a member of the university staff accompanied him to an open-air pool. At the edge of the pool he politely asked what the Dutch conventions were: turn left, turn right, straight lengths? After hearing that in the Netherlands we simply do whatever we like, he got into the water for a series of lengths in what the staff member called 'a powerful breaststroke'.

Forty years in America have not been without their effect. Sacks turned up wearing an orange baseball cap and fashionable trainers. But with his hat off and feet under the table, the man sitting across from me was unmistakably an Englishman by birth. There was no trace of an American accent. Sacks spoke gently and unassumingly, softly and with great precision.

In his afterword to *Uncle Tungsten*, Sacks writes that in 1997 a friend sent him a parcel containing a chemistry catalogue, a poster of the periodic system and a small bar of tungsten, which promptly fell to the floor with a 'resonant clonk' that immediately reminded him of his childhood. It was for him a Proustian moment that released memories of the time when he was obsessed with chemistry. But how could such a seemingly trivial event be the impetus for what would eventually become an autobiography?

Sacks: It was not anticipated when I was in my fifties, but around my sixtieth birthday I found memories from my boyhood were beginning to surface spontaneously, although this was also stimulated by a couple of opportunities. One was being asked to write an article on museums. For me, growing up in London, the museums – the Natural History Museum, the Geological Museum, the Science Museum – were much more important than any formal schooling. So I wrote about those and also an article on Humphry Davy, the chemist, and that brought me back to my own love of chemistry, my identification with Humphry Davy as a boy. This started the autobiographic impulse and once it started, it was like . . . er . . . urinating. I couldn't stop.

Draaisma: The autobiography is often taken to be the most intimate and personal of literary genres, but you seem to have turned it into something of a team effort, with all manner of assistance: your editor Kate Edgar, who provided you with magnets, minerals and crystals, your brothers and cousins, all helping you to dig up memories. It must have looked like a crowded excavation site.

Sacks: I can't think of a subject without wanting to enact it around me, so somewhat to Kate's distress and amusement, my apartment in New York is filled with metals, with magnets, with electrical machines which did duplicate many of my boyhood joys. Also, I still had many of my old chemistry and physics books and if I didn't have them, I went to some trouble with antiquarian booksellers to get them, not to see how they looked after the interval, but to try to stimulate the feeling they originally gave me. And sometimes memories were triggered by chance events. Finding myself on a bus in Mexico, with a couple who spoke Swiss-German, immediately transported me back almost fifty years to a bus in Lucerne, just after the war, which took us from the railway station to the hotel. That bus ride opened up many of the personal reminiscences in *Uncle*

Tungsten, as the tungsten bar opened up the more scientific reminiscences.

Draaisma: Reading about your intensely experimental boyhood and your passion for system and order, and upon learning that this boy would grow up to be a neurologist, one would expect a life spent in laboratories, perhaps a career as a brain cartographer.

Sacks: I always had fantasies of being a laboratory man, a neurophysiologist, but they worked out badly. There is a particularly terrible one, in 1965. I'd just finished my neurology training and I took a research year in neurochemistry and neuropathology. It was a disaster. I am very clumsy, I kept breaking apparatus, I lost some of my results, I lost specimens, and finally they said to me: 'Sacks, get out! You're a menace. Go and see patients, you won't do so much harm.' And when I did start seeing patients, in 1966, I found it a deep delight, of a quite different sort from the delight I found in chemistry. Among my first patients were people with migraine. Migraine is clearly a physiological attack, but why should people have it at particular times? I had to get them to keep calendars, I had to delve sometimes for unconscious determinants. It was the richness of psychic and physiological determination that fascinated me. The reason that I don't anticipate writing a second volume of autobiography any time soon is that after the age of fifteen there came a period in which I had not yet found my destiny, my voice. It seems unlikely that a length of tungsten will turn up for those years of my life. I'd be more likely to write a part three.

Draaisma: Did you find anything in neurology resembling the periodic table? Something with the same connotations of rigour and beauty and predictability?

Sacks: This boyhood chemistry was an ecstasy to me, it was what made sense and what had brought order after being rather traumatized in finding the world uncertain, capricious and chaotic. The periodic table was like an icon of order and predictability. I still carry it with me in my wallet. People often compare the genome to the periodic table, but in biology one has a sense of enormous contingency and of accident. In tungsten all atoms are the same – you know where you are with tungsten. In an animal population, variation is of the essence.

Draaisma: In *Uncle Tungsten* you write that Schubert's 'Nachtgesang' brings back the memory of your mother, singing slightly off-key, leaning over the piano, and you write that this memory comes with 'almost unbearable vividness'. Why 'unbearable'?

Sacks: That she's gone, that she's in the past, that one can't revisit the past, that she's dead, that that time is dead, but also I think there is an almost unbearable poignancy in a lot of Schubert's music. Years later, after my mother died, I could bear only Schubert.

Draaisma: Most people would have tried to avoid that music for a while.

Sacks: No. Perhaps it was a way of recreating her, not letting her go. She died in 1972. At the time I spent three months in London. I was completing *Awakenings*, living in a small apartment, and I would come down in the evening and read my mother the stories in *Awakenings*. Her reactions were very important to me. So 1972 was a very intense year for me, both in terms of loss and in terms of creation. I lost my mother, but I was given *Awakenings*. Years later, in 1993, my publisher wanted to celebrate an anniversary by getting his authors to describe one year each of the period since the publishing house was founded. The request reached me when I was in the car on the way to Canada. Friends, worried about me writing while I was driving, had given me a tape recorder and I started by speaking my memories of 1972 into it. When I had done 1972, I thought: why stop? – so I did 1973 and then 1974 and by the time I reached the Canadian border, about five hours later, I'd got up to 1989. I was afraid I would run out of tape, but in fact the latter years were getting shorter and shorter. The 1970s and early 1980s were very full and then I had less and less to say. The length decreased almost linearly. And why is that? Is it the repetition which enters one's life as one gets older? Does one store less and less? Or is it the intensity of youthful experiences? I can't really choose between those three hypotheses.

Draaisma: Has writing your autobiography in any way changed your personal or professional views on memory?

Sacks: I believed from the start that memories are based on something other than the simple reactivation of traces in the brain. Memories are reconstructions, and how you reconstruct them depends on your age, among other things. I did take into account that I'd have forgotten a great deal. But I was surprised that there were some memories, very vivid memories, that turned out to have been not so much reconstructed as completely fabricated, like the memory of the incendiary bomb. [In *Uncle Tungsten* Sacks describes two incidents involving bombs. During the Christmas holidays in 1940, which he was allowed to spend at home, a thousand-pounder landed in the neighbour's garden. Fortunately it failed to detonate, but the whole street had to be evacuated. Oliver, then aged seven, crept out of the house with his family, all of them walking as softly as they could to avoid making any vibrations that might set off the bomb. It was a strange procession: most people were still wearing pyjamas, the street was in pitch-darkness and everyone was holding a torch wrapped in red crêpe paper. The second bomb was an incendiary, a thermite bomb, and this one did detonate. Oliver's father rushed over with a stirrup pump and Oliver remembers how his brothers carried buckets of water over to him. 'But water seemed useless against this infernal fire – indeed, made it burn even more furiously. There was a vicious hissing and sputtering when the water hit the white-hot metal, and meanwhile the bomb was melting in its own casing and throwing blobs and jets of molten metal in all directions.'[4] The next day the lawn looked like a volcanic landscape.] A few months after the book was published, I spoke of these bombing incidents to my brother Michael. He immediately confirmed the first bombing incident, saying, 'I remember it exactly as you described it'. But regarding the second bombing, he said, 'You never saw it. You weren't there'. I was staggered at Michael's words. How could he dispute a memory I would not hesitate to swear to in a court of law and had never doubted as real? 'What do you mean?' I objected. 'I can see the bomb in my mind's eye now, Pop with his pump, and Marcus and David with their buckets of water. How could I see it so clearly if I wasn't there?' 'You never saw it,' Michael repeated. 'We were both away at Braefield at the time. But David [their older brother] wrote us a letter about it. A very vivid, dramatic letter. You were enthralled by it.' Clearly, I had not only been enthralled, but must have constructed the scene in my mind, from David's words, and then taken it over, appropriated it, and taken it for a memory of my own.

After Michael said this, I tried to compare the two memories – the primary one, whose direct experiential stamp was not in doubt, with the constructed or secondary one. With the first incident, I could feel myself into the body of the little boy, shivering in his thin pyjamas – it was December, and I was terrified – and because of my shortness compared to the big adults all around me, I had to crane my head upwards to see their faces. The second image, of the thermite bomb, was equally clear, it seemed to me – very vivid, detailed and concrete. I tried to persuade myself that it had a different quality from the first, that it bore evidences of its appropriation from someone else's experience and its translation from verbal description into image. But although I now know, intellectually, that this memory was 'false', secondary, appropriated, translated, it still seems to me as real, as intensely my own, as before.

Another memory has stayed with Sacks from that same short period at home, this time an embarrassing one. He was crazy about Greta, the dachshund, who greeted him with delight when he arrived home, rolling around and squirming with joy. Nevertheless:

> ... one of my first acts, that winter, was to imprison her in the freezing coal bin in the yard outside, where her pitiful whimperings and barkings could not be heard. She was missed after a while, and I was asked, we were all asked, when we had last seen her, whether we had any idea where she was. I thought of her – hungry, cold, imprisoned, perhaps dying in the coal bin outside – but said nothing. It was only toward evening that I admitted what I had done, and Greta was fetched, almost frozen, from the bin. My father was furious and gave me 'a good hiding' and stood me in a corner for the rest of the day.[5]

At the time, as a seven-year-old, he would not have been able to explain what had got into him, but now, looking back, Sacks writes: 'It was surely a message, a symbolic act of some kind, trying to draw my parents' attention to *my* coal bin, Braefield, my misery and helplessness there.'[6]

Draaisma: In *Uncle Tungsten* you write very candidly about your first orgasm, and about memories you find embarrassing even today. Would you say that this may be age-related as well? Could you have written about such things when you were in your forties or fifties?

Sacks: Each time I see a dachshund I think of poor Greta . . . I write partly to make a confession, but also partly to seek forgiveness, including forgiveness from myself. I think of that in almost religious terms, of judgment and accusation and reconciliation. I think I did find that many painful and unresolved matters from childhood, including the cruelty to the dog, were not excused but made comprehensible by writing about it. I've heard people say that psychoanalysis may be bad for a writer because it will defuse the memories, but I almost thought of *Uncle Tungsten* as part of the ongoing analytic process, which is about bringing things out.

Draaisma: You've been in psychoanalysis since 1966.

Sacks: I started my psychoanalysis in January 1966. My therapist and I, we've grown old together . . . He has always felt that the Braefield years were the most significant, in a negative way. I fear sometimes the negative has psychically almost killed my brother

Michael and I thought it might kill me. It's too easy to speak in terms of 'compensation'; perhaps I would have fallen passionately in love with chemistry and science anyhow. I do know that when I'm distressed I like to read botany or physics to get away from it.

Draaisma: Do you ever reflect on the course your life has taken from a professional point of view?

Sacks: I was reflecting on this in a very melancholy way, in the train coming to Groningen. I was feeling rather ill and I was in a dark mood. I had just been reading the autobiography by Eric Kandel [a physiologist who made his name with measurements of electrical activity in single nerve cells] and I contrasted that satisfying, logical and linear life with what I often feel is my own life. The life of a doctor is different from that of a scientist. I am very dependent on accident, on people knocking on the door, phoning me, writing me a letter, which may set me off. So I had no clear feeling of a career, of a trajectory. But I think as the works multiply, perhaps they begin to circumscribe some perspective, some sensibility, some intellectual orientation which is of value. I get very moved sometimes when students come up to me and say 'I read your book when I was in high school and that made me want to be a doctor'.

I dare to say, in my eighth decade, that somehow I may be able to bring things together, more than I have. People always say: 'Sacks, where is your theory?', but I'm not a person for general theory. I will provide stories, case histories, examples, which will be the material.

Draaisma: And now you have so many honorary degrees to your name, memberships of prestigious societies, honorary fellowships, literary and scientific awards . . .

Sacks: I think I have been a good doctor to my patients. A couple of days ago I saw one of my elderly patients; I felt I had listened sympathetically and carefully to her, made clever suggestions, and I came back with the feeling I had been a good neurological workman. My parents, who were good doctors, would recognize that I'm a good doctor too. They might have mixed feelings about other things. I remember all too vividly, in 1970, when *Migraine*, my first book, came out, that my father came into my room, at six in the morning, grey, trembling, holding *The Times* and said: 'You're in the paper!' *The Times* actually had written a beautiful article about the book, calling it balanced, brilliant, authoritative. But to my father none of this mattered, it was merely the scandal of being in the papers, of having become visible. This was partly a personal thing with him, but also a matter of medical ethics, which was strong and said there were various forbidden things, all beginning with A: adultery was one of them, alcohol and addiction were others, and one of them was advertisement. My father thought it was wrong of me to have brought my name before a larger public. And I incorporated that view. To this day I have two persistent Freudian errors: I tend to misread 'publish' as 'punish' and 'portray' as 'betray', so first I had to struggle with what I felt was the impropriety of making anything public that was confidential, and secondly with what was the fear of exploiting or exposing my patients.

Draaisma: Your father lived until 1990. Did his attitude towards your work change?

Sacks: Yes, it did. My father did become more benign and, perhaps, proud of me. But I was also proud of him. He was a humble man. He was actually too humble. In England there are almost two strata in medicine: the general practitioners, the workmen, and then there are the specialists who are felt to be of higher calibre, socially and intellectually higher. But my father was an extraordinary diagnostician. He was always coming up with things that specialists had missed. And he worked very, very hard. When he was ninety they said to him 'please stop doing house calls' and he said: 'I'll stick with the house calls, forget everything else.' He lived to be almost ninety-five. He started as a GP in his early twenties, so he put seventy-plus years of experience into those house calls.

Draaisma: You left England when you were just twenty-seven.

Sacks: I think I partly left England to get away from my parents and to get away from what I felt was a tight and rigid medical hierarchy. My brother Michael went to Australia. Both of us wanted space, moral space, intellectual space, physical space, and we both carry resentments and ambivalences toward our parents. There is an angry subtext to *Uncle Tungsten*, but as I get older I begin to see that they were hard workers and that they did their best. It wasn't the easiest of times and I wasn't the easiest of sons. I must have been a hard son at times. I also think that I made them feel that in some sense I'd got beyond them, and that both excited and frightened me and I think it frightened them.

Draaisma: So in a sense you were a good son by leaving.

Sacks: That's a way of putting it.

CHAPTER SEVEN

Wisdom in hindsight

Memories are about the past. Whether you are thinking back to a reprimand you received from a teacher forty years ago or trying to recall what happened last night, memories refer to something that lies behind you. And because the past is fixed once and for all – what's done is done – if you notice that a memory has changed, then you will have a natural tendency to regard it as unreliable. This is all too easy to explain: we see memories as recordings of what we experienced, as things we have entered in a register. If discrepancies emerge in our bookkeeping over time, then we feel intuitively that we cannot rely on our memories.

In fact, however, this is a case of our intuition falling prey to a tempting syllogism. The premises are correct: memories are about the past and the past does not change. But we draw the wrong conclusion. Every memory makes a connection between two poles in time. What you remember may have happened yesterday or half a century ago; the fact that you remember it is a present-day fact. Remembering something is an act that happens now. When you use your powers of recall, not only does something of your younger self appear in the present but, conversely, elements of your feelings and thoughts in the present end up in the memory. Memories are not files that, after you've looked at them, go back into the archives in precisely the same condition as when you took them out. Using them changes them. Furthermore, the memory of one and the same event can feel different depending on your mood at that moment. The memory, writes Dutch novelist Nicolaas Matsier, 'is like a cook serving up a meal made from whatever was available. But it's never the same meal'.[1]

In the year he turned fifty, historian Wim Willems, born and bred in The Hague, started to chronicle his childhood memories. They cover roughly the late 1950s and the 1960s. He tells of the lodger they had, old Mr de Graaf, former coachman to Queen Wilhelmina and Prince Hendrik. Wim occasionally went into the lodger's room, which smelled of paraffin. 'There was the smell of stale smoke and something else, which I couldn't identify at the time but now realize must have been the fumes of Dutch gin.'[2] This is precisely, in microcosm, how an experience from the past is brought into the present, with an interpretation that relies on present-day knowledge. Willems remembers an alcoholic who did not yet exist for young Wim.

There is a second intuition about our memories that does not stand close examination. In life we are aware of an asymmetry that works to the benefit of old age, or so we are inclined to think: a person of sixty knows what it is like to be twenty, whereas a person of twenty cannot know what it is like to be sixty. We all have the feeling that the twenty-year-old we once were has left traces of his or her experiences in our memories and that these can be found again in the midst of all the traces from later years, rather in the way that the young tree is still there in the old tree, beneath all the later growth rings. We think we can remember enough to reconstruct the twenty-year-old. Unfortunately this is too simplistic. Not only did many of the memories of the twenty-year-old vanish long ago, what we now have, all these years later, are at best memories of memories – a very different matter. Memories are selective, incomplete and coloured. This is also the case with memories of memories, but they present the additional problem that they make you realize you may no longer have access to the original memory, because you cannot possibly recover the perspective you had at the time. I remember a fierce row with my father about being obliged to go to confirmation classes when I was about sixteen. I also remember that for a long time I looked back on that dispute with a sense of triumph. I was extremely satisfied with my arguments and my sarcastic comments on the principle of baptismal vows. Nowadays it is impossible for me to remember our exchange of words as it was in the original memory. When I think back on it, that atmosphere of triumph has been replaced by shame – shame at how impervious I was to the things that motivated him and the aspirations he had for his children, shame at my sarcasm, shame at my self-importance. The original scene is still there, but it can no longer be recalled as I once remembered it, and in that sense it has been forgotten. This kind of forgetting is not simply a matter of traces being wiped away; rather it seems as if we no longer have any access to some traces, and that this has to do with changes in our lives that alter our perspective on the past.

The writing of an autobiography or memoir activates the same two poles in time as remembering. The things that need to be described are in the past, whereas the writing happens in the present. But something else follows on from this contact. The memories that are recalled must be set down on paper. Memories that, as memories, could have remained what they were – a smell, a feeling, a mood, an image – now have to be put into words and, for the sake of readability, made part of a story. Perhaps writers are more painfully aware than anyone that language is not only a necessary step towards the reader but also a step away from memory. Writers know they are creating worlds out of words, rather than describing, and that the slightest nuances in the way they express themselves displace things in those worlds. There are autobiographies in which this has become almost the main theme: the awareness of putting a life story down on paper that could have been told differently, hard as the writer may try to describe memories as truthfully as possible. Like biographies, autobiographies present not lives but versions of lives.

When Günter Grass was in his late seventies, he wrote *Peeling the Onion*, an autobiography covering roughly the first thirty years of his life. It was published in 2006. On almost every page we can feel the unease the writer experiences about his contact with his earlier self. There are two reasons for this, and Grass, a sensitive observer of that younger self, continually hints at them. The first is simply the absence of memories of much of what he thought and felt as an infant, boy and adolescent. Not everything has gone, but there are so many voids, lacunae and blanks that he writes with great hesitation about the boy he once was. He prefers to take refuge in the third person: 'Books have always been his gap in the fence.' Or even in the interrogative: 'In what direction was he spooling his thread?'³ Later there is a schoolboy, a recruit, a trainee tank gunner, a war casualty and a mineworker with his name, all five of them with a mental life that has become largely inaccessible. Writing about 'the youth I am trying to imagine as an early damaged edition of myself',⁴ Grass calls on his powers of empathy more than on his memory. As to the motives of all those past namesakes, he remembers little as he approaches eighty. Only after his arrival at the art academy in Düsseldorf does the third person gradually give way to the first. The protagonist is well into his twenties by then, and in the ten years in which Grass developed into the writer he would eventually become – *The Tin Drum* was published in 1959 – more of a connection seems to develop between him and the subject he is writing about. The autobiography can therefore continue more consistently in the first person.

At least as unsettling are the memories that do remain. At the Conradinum gymnasium in Danzig, where Grass grew up, he had a friend called Wolfgang Heinrichs. Grass vividly remembers how the boy managed to reel off not just the victories of the German advance but the defeats, which he claimed were considerable. 'You haven't a clue about what really went on up there in the north. There were heavy losses! Damned heavy!'[5] It does not occur to the boys to ask how he knows this. Shortly after the summer holidays, when Wolfgang suddenly stops coming to school, everyone is surprised, but no one thinks about it for long, young Günter included; he barely notices. Fifty years later, shortly after German unification, Grass and his wife Ute visit her native island of Hiddensee and hear that a certain Heinrichs lives there who swears that Grass and he were once in the same class at school. Grass visits him and only then does he hear the story of the boy's disappearance. Wolfgang's father was an anti-Fascist, and in the early autumn of 1940 he was arrested by the Gestapo and sent to a concentration camp. The boy's despairing mother killed herself. Wolfgang and his sister were sent to stay with their grandmother in the countryside, 'far enough away to have been forgotten by their schoolmates'.[6] The father was eventually released to serve in a penal battalion whose job it was to clear mines on the Russian front. It was nicknamed the Ascension Commando. He defected to the Russians, came back to Danzig with the Red Army and found his children. Wolfgang grew up in the GDR.

Writing about Wolfgang Heinrichs as a school chum aged thirteen, Grass cannot ignore what he now knows about the course of Wolfgang's life then and later. Above all he cannot free himself from an intense sense of shame at not having missed him at the time, at not even having asked where he had got to. His earlier self silently accepted the boy's disappearance, 'so that now, as I peel the onion, my silence pounds in my ears'.[7]

He has other, similar memories. A common factor is that they point to what happened fifty or sixty years ago but are both charged and illuminated by what followed, and this has turned them into different memories. They are no longer available in their original form.

Do we underestimate the extent to which memories change and vanish? It seems probable that we do. We rarely make notes about what we think and believe. Even people who keep journals generally write more about what happened than about their underlying motives, about what they did rather than why they did it. The continual rewriting of our personal history passes unnoticed. Our memories repeatedly construct a different past, even though they are rarely caught doing so. Occasionally circumstances arise in which the one can be laid next to the other, the earlier version next to the later, and then all that deleting, supplementing and revising acquires a visibility that makes us realize how many changes take place without ever coming to our attention.

Two American psychologists were given access to answers to the California Test of Personality provided by almost 500 students in 1944.[8] It is a test that enquires about relationships in the family, at school and with friends, aiming to capture characteristics such as self-reliance and a sense of personal worth, and the development of social skills. The students were on average nineteen years old at the time. In 1969 a great many from the original group – now in their mid-forties – were invited to take the test again. More than fifty agreed to do so. They responded to the test twice, once to give answers according to their current personality and relationships, and a second time to give the answers they thought they had given in 1944. Comparison of the scores shows that the characteristics themselves remained relatively constant: those who had a considerable sense of personal worth and self-reliance at the age of nineteen still had those character traits twenty-five years later; those who had described themselves as socially isolated did so again in the 1969 test. The real surprise lay in the results of their attempts to reproduce the answers given in 1944. There were huge differences between the actual 1944 answers and the remembered 1944 answers. Now in their mid-forties, the respondents had clearly lost touch with the nineteen-year-olds they once were. Generally speaking, their remembered answers were more negative than they had been in 1944: more conflict, less self-confidence, poorer social skills. It seems as if people in middle age will remember an adolescent who is unhappier than they actually thought themselves to be at the time.

Another experiment shows even more tellingly that the memory re-edits the past. In 1962 Daniel Offer, a psychiatrist in

Chicago, began a long-term study into the psychological development of a group of teenagers who were approaching adulthood. He interviewed seventy-three young men in their first year of high school – aged about thirteen – and followed them for several years after they left school.[9] Thirty-five years later, in 1997, he contacted them again and found almost seventy prepared to be interviewed.[10] Each interview lasted for more than four hours, with part of the time spent on the same questions as were asked in 1962. There have been a number of studies of this kind. They make clear that beliefs and convictions are subject to considerable changes over the course of a lifetime. But Offer gave a fascinating twist to his research by issuing his interviewees with one unusual instruction. They were asked to imagine themselves as once again the young men they were in 1962 and to give answers that would fit with the way they thought then. One of the questions in 1962 had been: Who is your mother's favourite, you or one of your brothers or sisters? Now the question was: When you were thirteen, who did you think was your mother's favourite? The man of forty-eight had to call up in himself the thirteen-year-old he once was and try to answer according to the truth of thirty-five years ago.

The interviews covered all kinds of things: their thoughts and experiences as thirteen-year-olds, their self-image and personality, how they regarded sexuality and girls, their friends and hobbies, their position in the family and in class, their upbringing, their parents' characters and their feelings about religion.

Looking back over a distance of thirty-five years, it turns out, does something dramatic to your memory. A few points at random. To the question 'Who do you think is your mother's favourite, you or one of the other children?' 30 per cent of the men answered: 'Me' – twice as many as had done so in 1962. In other words a great many of the middle-aged men had become their mother's favourite child in retrospect. Thirty-five years earlier, 70 per cent of the teenage boys thought they took after their fathers more than their mothers; among forty-eight-year-olds it was fifty–fifty. Many of the questions revealed a discrepancy between then and now that amounted to a doubling or halving. The middle-aged men were twice as likely to describe their upbringing by their fathers as strict. Which of your parents takes or took most of the decisions at home? There was a substantial shift in favour of the mother. The 'yes' to the question of whether you were sometimes smacked at home fell from 82 to 33 per cent.

Much of the existing research into autobiographical memory concentrates on the reliability of memories. In some situations the degree of reliability is of great importance, in witness statements for instance, but for many memories quite different factors matter more. Memories do indeed have a tendency to change over the course of a lifetime, but the fact that memories change is perhaps the least interesting aspect. More important is: how do they change and why?

Take those fathers who after thirty-five years were twice as often regarded as strict. Perhaps the forty-eight-year-olds were comparing their 1950s fathers to the 1980s fathers they themselves became. Perhaps they saw themselves as one of those 'I'm my son's best friend' fathers. By comparison their own fathers became stricter in their memories than they were at the time. I can see a parallel here with black-and-white television. Until colour television arrived, no one had a black-and-white television set. You simply had a television. In a philosophical sense, black-and-white television came after colour television. Similarly, many of those thirteen-year-old boys did not have strict fathers; they became strict only after the arrival of more lenient conventions of upbringing. It is the same effect as that which can cause a person to remember an austere childhood in retrospect that was not experienced as such at the time.

What counts as truth here? What counts as dependability? These are the wrong questions. Our memories are full of black-and-white television sets. The fact that you remember your father and mother differently when you are forty-eight from the way you called them to mind when you were thirteen does not mean that your memories, those of the present day or those of the past, are 'unreliable'. Rather it shows that your memories provide you with a past in which people and events can change their significance. The real asymmetry between being young and being old is that those who are old have far more experience of the fact that, as we age, the past turns out to be just as unsettled as the future. This might be described as a particularly interesting form of wisdom in hindsight.

CHAPTER EIGHT

The nostalgia factory

Shortly after the Second World War, Lyckele de Jong from Oudeschoot in the Dutch province of Friesland emigrates to New Zealand to build a new life for himself. As he is leaving, his father slips a pair of Fenland speed skates into his bag: if there are streams in that distant country or stretches of flooded land and it starts to freeze, he says, you'll go crazy if you don't have any skates. One Sunday in July, in the middle of the New Zealand winter, Lyckele wakes up to a frozen world. The sago palms are covered in hoar frost. Temperatures clearly got down to well below zero overnight. It is Lyckele's first day off after months of slaving away at the Roxburgh dam. He rents a horse, takes a bag of oats with him and some sandwiches, and heads off between the flanks of the inhospitable Otago Mountains. After riding for several hours he sees a bluish sheen in the valley below him. He makes his way down. Before long he is standing next to a lake as big as the Tjeukemeer. He looks around, stamps on the ice here and there, determines that it is at least five inches thick and puts on his skates. At first he stays close to the shore, accompanied by the ominous cracking and booming of untrodden ice, before finally letting himself go, hands at his back, gliding across the endless surface.

Then something happens that Lyckele still regards as a miracle even half a century later. At the far end of the lake, there in the middle of nowhere, he sees a couple of dots moving. He skates towards them and soon finds himself shaking hands with three men, a farm labourer from Akmaryp, a builder from Huizum and a butcher's boy from Sneek. All are using traditional skates from Friesland, designed for speed and distance. At the other end of the world they spend the rest of the afternoon skimming across the lake in formation.

We are familiar with vicarious embarrassment. Is there such a thing as vicarious nostalgia? Because nostalgia is what I feel every time I read this story. More than anything it comes from those brief snatches of 'home' that pop up now and then in this far-off life of Lyckele's. First of all those skates, of course, slipped into his bag by his father. But there is also the home that resonates in 'as big as the Tjeukemeer', in place names like Sneek and Akmaryp, in the booming of the virgin ice and the style of skating, with hands clasped at the small of the back. If nostalgia can reside in movement, in the sensation of freezing wind on your skin, the hardness of ice, the hoarse scrape of the blades, the unexpected company of other men from Friesland, then what Lyckele felt on that lake was nostalgia.

His story was written up by Hylke Speerstra in *Cruel Paradise*.[1] Speerstra travelled to meet emigrants who left the Netherlands shortly after the Second World War. Boarding ship in Rotterdam, they took long sea voyages to destinations chosen for them by the three main emigration agencies, each of which was allied to one of the church denominations in which they had grown up: Calvinists went westwards to Canada and the United States (mostly to Michigan), Catholics went to New Zealand and Australia, and members of the Dutch Reformed Church went to South Africa. By the time the great tide of emigration began to ebb in the mid-1960s, half a million Dutch people had emigrated. Sometimes, because of that same division by denomination, they ended up in small communities of fellow believers, but more often they lived in an unfamiliar environment, coping with an uprooted existence that was no less tarnished by poverty than the life they had left behind. For work and housing they depended on the people who had always lived there, or on earlier emigrants. There was hardly anything in the way of a social safety net. Often the man of the family would leave first, and only after he had a roof over his head and a secure job could his fiancée, wife or children follow him out. Integration with the local population was not a matter of rights or duties but of simple necessity, learning the language a question of survival. Forenames that had been passed down from generation to generation, representing family ties with ancestors and nephews and nieces, were exchanged for names that sounded vaguely similar but were easier to use. Jeen became James, Sytske became Sally, Rinze became Ray and, in Brazil, Foppe, rather small in stature, went through life from then on as Fopinho. Many of their stories have a special glow from having been told by people older than the parents who watched them leave.

Lyckele – now called Nick – succeeded in building a good life for himself. After a year he was able to bring over his fiancée, Aly ten Boom, who found a job in the fruit-growing trade. They bought a run-down farm, almost went under as the result of a rabbit plague, recovered by shooting rabbits for the bounty, managed to withstand the vicissitudes of fate, produced three strapping sons and now, fifty years later, have retired to a large farm in the mild climate of northern New Zealand. Aly says that in the first few years her husband sometimes felt homesick; Lyckele himself prefers to say that he took a while to adjust. In those days he might suddenly wake in the middle of the night having dreamed he was back home:

Sometimes I'd be up to my ears in that terribly cold winter during the war, and then I'd find myself on the old Church Lane tramping back to town. My hands would be so cold that I'd be all bent over. I must've been about twelve when, at the end of the path where there are all kinds of factories now, I met Gabe Westra. He saw me shivering and hollered: 'Hey, aren't you one of the kids of Lyckele and Jantsje? You may hold my warm pipe for a while. That'll warm your hands in no time.'[2]

Aly concluded from this: 'Young emigrants dream about their childhood, old immigrants about the early years of their new life. That way you dream two lives.'[3]

So much nostalgia. In retrospect the emigrants are more astonished by that than by anything else: they left because of poverty, housing shortages and unemployment yet were eaten up by homesickness. The post-war wave of emigration from the Netherlands was composed not of teachers, preachers and doctors but of plodding farm boys, agricultural labourers and hard-working tradesmen. Many decisions to emigrate were inspired by a longing to leave, to get out and go somewhere new, which sounds like the opposite of nostalgia, but once they had left, one in five felt such a longing for home that they went back. Those who stayed – and Speerstra spoke only to them – had to deal with their homesickness as best they could. It raises its head in every single chapter of *Cruel Paradise*, sometimes as a feeling that tugged and nagged and dissipated only when children were born, sometimes as a pain that grew worse with the years. 'At first you hardly feel it,' says Anna Postma, who emigrated to Canada with her husband Nies. 'But then suddenly you don't have an appetite anymore, and then you can't sleep anymore. Still later you suffer the consequences of that, and at last it seeps through your whole system and settles in your marrow. Finally, in the last phase, it attacks you mentally, and you go crazy. You die from it.'[4] For Anna it ended in a nervous breakdown that saw her hospitalized. Her children were cared for by other Dutch emigrants, so within a year of their arrival the family was split up. It would take years for the homesickness to subside. With Nies, by contrast, it surfaced in old age. Despite eight trips to Friesland and walks through his native village of Tzum, he became depressed and eventually died of a heart complaint.

So homesickness can strike twice. In the early years after emigration it sometimes pulled families apart, the wife wanting to return and the man to stay. Some women hoped their homesickness would ease once a baby came, but then as young mothers they were ambushed by a desperate desire to show the child to their parents. Fifty years later, nostalgia can still divide families, when one wants to return to the native country while the other wants to stay with the children and grandchildren. The intervening half-century has reversed the roles: now it is usually the man who wants to go back, not his wife. It seems that for men, 'home' is where they were born, whereas for women it is where their children were born.

Sometimes homesickness lasts even beyond death. In Melbourne, Speerstra spoke to Liesbeth Niemarkt, widow of Wiebe Boersma. They emigrated in 1952 with their three sons. Four years later they were back in Leeuwarden, because Wiebe felt homesick. After a few years in Leeuwarden he felt homesick again, this time for Australia. They applied to emigrate a second time. Wiebe's nostalgia would ultimately send them back and forth another three times. Finally they stayed in Australia, but shortly before he died, Wiebe began to fret. He wanted his ashes to go back to Friesland, to be scattered over the Pikmeer and the surrounding pastures. As soon as he had been cremated, the package of ash started its long journey. After six months aboard ship it was lost during unloading, found again, and delivered to distant nephews and nieces who kept it in the hall for some time before finally in desperation giving it to the manager of a cemetery in Leeuwarden. Speerstra writes: 'The man who appeared in the door said: "I'll take care of it."'[5]

Those emigration agencies were nostalgia factories. But in the era when the emigrants left, nostalgia arose closer to home too, in barracks and sanatoria, in seminaries and boarding schools, in prisons and hospitals, in all those institutions that take people from home and detain them, permanently or temporarily, with nothing but their memories. Of the four Dutch dissertations on the subject of nostalgia, two have their origins in barracks, or to be more precise in military hospitals and psychiatric clinics.[6] This is no accident; conscription was a formidable producer of nostalgia, which can lead to illness and psychological harm. In the Netherlands (as in France: *nostalgie permanente*) nostalgia is official grounds for finding a person unfit for military service. Now that troops are sent on peace missions in far-off countries, articles about it appear regularly in Dutch journals about military medicine. They include reports of research into the socio-demographic symptoms of soldiers suffering from homesickness, the circumstances that pave the way for it and the psychopathology of those who succumb.

Nostalgia is an early example of what might almost be called a medical invention.[7] In 1688 a Swiss doctor called Johannes Hofer wrote his thesis about the case of a young man from Bern who went to study at university in Basel and soon felt consumed by a longing for home. It made him ill. He lost his appetite, shedding weight noticeably, and eventually his physical condition deteriorated to such an extent that there were fears for his life. The pharmacist, who had tried one medicine after another in vain, advised him simply to return to Bern. That certainly helped. Merely knowing his return was imminent brought about a turn for the better and by the time he was halfway to Bern the student had fully recovered. As a name for the illness Hofer chose the Swiss dialect word *Heimweh* (homesickness) and 'translated' it into Greek. From *nostos*, homecoming, and *algia*, pain, he derived the word 'nostalgia', a neologism that has been taken up by many other languages and is used to this day, although few remember its medical background.

Hofer described the cause of the illness in terms derived from Descartes, the originator of an understanding of neurology that was regarded as authoritative at the time. Descartes believed that nerves were hollow tubes that contained a gas-like substance capable of stretching them. When a person thought a lot about home, calling up remembered images that were stored away in the brain, the nerve fibres linked to those images became so stretched that eventually home was all he or she could think about. Every association, wherever in the patient's brain it started out, ended up at 'home'.

Although Hofer described only two cases, in an account of no more than eleven pages, the response from the medical world was overwhelming. All over Europe cases of 'nostalgia' were discovered, a potentially deadly sickness that always took the same course, involving weight loss and apathy. Theodore Zwinger, a colleague of Hofer and a fellow Swiss, saw nostalgia above all as a disorder originating in the memory. In 1720 he wrote that in soldiers fighting in foreign lands who amused themselves by singing songs from home, a fatal process would take root: the songs brought up more and more memories of home until eventually it was all they could think about and in the worst cases they succumbed to the dreaded nostalgia.[8] With armies consisting largely of mercenaries, it was army doctors who most often encountered nostalgia. In the nineteenth century the illness sometimes reached epidemic proportions during campaigns. Until Napoleonic times, abnormalities in the brain were discovered during autopsies performed on soldiers who had died of nostalgia.[9] It was not until the twentieth century that nostalgia shifted from being considered an organic disorder to a psychological complaint. It was psychiatry that brought about the switch.

By far the most renowned dissertation on nostalgia is by psychiatrist and philosopher Karl Jaspers. It was published in 1909 under the title *Heimweh und Verbrechen* (*Nostalgia and Crime*).[10] In it he presents a series of case studies, mainly of young women who, having recently gone into service for the first time, committed serious crimes out of homesickness. Some strangled or poisoned a child in their care; others tried to kill their mistresses. To take one case out of many, a girl not even ten years old went into service as a nursemaid. She longed for her mother, but her mistress forbade her to go home. She ran away, but was brought back by her mother and the next day she strangled a child she was looking after. No one suspected her, and the three-year-old brother of the dead boy remained in her care. The next day she set fire to the house, thinking: if the child dies and the house burns down, there will be no further need for a nursemaid. But her arson attempt failed. In the end she took a blanket, spread it over the child and sat on it until the little boy died. Jaspers and his contemporaries collected dozens of such cases, the vast majority of which are tales of intense homesickness leading to arson. One detail illustrates the despair of all those children longing for home: a girl of fifteen missed her grandmother so much that she took a glowing coal out of the fire, carried it to the barn in her bare hands and lay it on the hay.

Jaspers' dissertation was not a study of the subject in the modern sense: there are no questionnaires, no statistics, no tables, no models, no flow charts of causal, facilitating and mediating factors. Yet the reader is left with the feeling that there is not very much to add to his observations. The symptoms he describes are loss of appetite, compulsive thoughts of home, longing to return home, apathy, melancholy and sleeplessness. He also notes the counterproductive effects of home. After the young maids and nursemaids had visited home for a few days, their nostalgia became worse. Many of their crimes were committed shortly after a trip home, or after a father or mother had come to visit. Girls who were allowed to take a sister with them were no less homesick than those who went into service on their own. Illness or injury intensified their nostalgia. Distraction sometimes helped, especially physical work, but activities that left them alone with their thoughts, such as reading, brought the nostalgia back. Homesickness lay in wait for them at the edges of the night, when they were unable to get to sleep or woke up very early. Even girls who were better off in service than they had been at home were struck down by it; better to be at home without anything to eat than to be away from home and unable to eat for nostalgia.

For a long time after Jaspers' book was published, the literature on the subject of nostalgia was forensically oriented, fading away as the crimes committed in nostalgia's name – or, rather, the specific type of perpetrator – ceased to exist. There is room for an interesting if rather gruesome book about the rise and fall of crimes of nostalgia: how homesickness mainly affected young girls who had grown up in families that had little contact with life in town or in bourgeois circles; how going into service, given the limited means of communication and transport of the time, meant a complete break with home; how girls ended up in families where personal relationships were very different from those to which they were accustomed; how, in short, a handful of demographic and social factors conspired to produce crimes like arson and infanticide.

Modern nostalgia is measured according to various scales, such as the Utrecht Homesickness Scale (UHS), developed by Tony van

Vliet.[11] Almost fifty situations are listed, and the sufferer can indicate on a five-point scale the degree to which these have occurred over the past four weeks: crying fits, dreams about the past, missing a partner, searching for familiar faces, missing familiar food, missing home, friends or family, longing for the comforts and company of home, endlessly thinking of home, feeling lonely, or feeling unable to cope with their new circumstances. Van Vliet gained his PhD in social sciences with this project, in which the medical jargon, with its pathology, diagnosis, symptoms and therapy, is replaced by that of the psychologist: stress, trauma, attachment, introversion, cognition, neurosis. The case studies have given way to questionnaires. The results are expressed in terms of correlations between homesickness scores and variables such as personality, situational factors such as distance from home, and social support, coping strategies and demographic factors. There are no cases of arson prompted by nostalgia in this dissertation, just as in Jaspers' work you will search in vain for holiday homesickness, whether of the 'current' or the 'anticipated' variety (some people feel homesick even before they leave).

Over the past ten years, several studies on nostalgia have appeared.[12] Here are some of their findings. There are no differences between men and women when it comes to susceptibility, but there is a personality profile: if a person is rigid by nature with a tendency to introversion, the risk of homesickness is greater. Dependency and a lack of self-respect also seem to increase the chances of contracting the disorder. Nostalgia increases with the distance from home and the length of time spent away. Forced removal from home, as for example in the case of a child moving house, leads to more homesickness than a voluntary move. There seems to be a gentle gradient: the younger you are, the greater the risk of homesickness, so it occurs more often in boarding-school children than among university students, although the degree to which the move is voluntary may impact upon the results in such cases. There seems to be hardly any mitigating effect associated with friends making the same move at the same time. Nostalgia may be one of a number of depressive symptoms, but it should not be confused with depression: homesickness can quickly be cured by a ticket home, whereas depression cannot. So if you are slightly withdrawn by nature, contemplative, if you have never been very outgoing, if you are not very socially adept and do not make friends easily, if you found your partner at a young age and have always stayed with him or her, if you prefer to know beforehand what you are getting into and dislike having to adjust your plans, if you are not keen on improvisation, and if despite all this you let yourself be sent a long way away more or less against your will, for example because it suits your employer, to a place where you have little to distract you and little social support, then the almost inevitable result is homesickness, profound nostalgia to the point of illness. You will probably very soon be back.

Four or five of these contributing factors form an ominous constellation over the heads of refugees and asylum-seekers, who are forced to leave home and family by danger, poverty, war or the threat of starvation. They end up in social and financial relationships that are entirely foreign to them. They have come a long way, and not only geographically. The opportunities to communicate with home are limited. There is little to distract them. The language is unfamiliar. They find themselves dependent on others, which erodes their self-esteem. Everything that was once expected of those who emigrated and was often such an effective weapon in the battle against homesickness – roll up your sleeves, learn the language, look for work, find your way in a new society – is forbidden to or made difficult for people caught up in the asylum process. Even those who departed out of a longing to be elsewhere will not escape intense nostalgia. Now that conscription has ended in most Western countries and girls are no longer sent into service at the age of ten, centres for asylum-seekers can be regarded as the nostalgia factories of our day.

In 1846 the French doctor Louis Alexandre Hippolyte Leroy-Dupré predicted that nostalgia would soon cease to exist. 'Cerebral nostalgia becomes rarer each day thanks to rapid communications which modern industry is beginning to establish among peoples who will soon be nothing more than one big family.'[13] Steam power, railways, packet boats that were setting up scheduled services, the telegraph – the shrinking world of 1846 would drive out nostalgia as a sickness. But despite the additional advantages of air travel, radio and the telephone, the Frisians who emigrated a century after Dupré's prophecy proved he was wrong. Many of the Canadian, Australian and American family doctors who were confronted with all that Frisian nostalgia in their consulting rooms in the 1950s advised their patients to go home and come back once they were cured. It seems they had not read Jaspers, who could have told them that such a move would be counterproductive. Their 'home' had changed in the meantime, so they wandered lost and uprooted in both worlds. Emigrants who had visited their old homes noticed that once they were back in the new country their nostalgia soon flared again. Baker Jochum Velstra of Ouwedijk near St Jacobiparochie, who had left for Australia in 1951, was advised by his doctor to buy a return ticket to Ouwedijk. One of his sons said: 'Six times our father made a return trip to Friesland in his battle with homesickness. Never with our mother, who was also struggling, but always alone. In short, all our hard-earned money evaporated into the stratosphere between Port Kembla and Ouwedijk through the jet engines. Still, the man worked in the bakery, and we baked bread that was soaked in his tears.'[14]

In old age, many emigrants experience a revival of the nostalgia that seemed quiescent for forty or fifty years. In a retirement home near Melbourne, Mrs Snijder says that her husband Willem still sees his parents, brothers and sisters waving to him from the jetty. 'Then he becomes melancholy, and I say: "Watch out my boy, we don't want any trouble with homesickness in our old age. We've had enough of that already!"' But there is nothing Willem can do about it: 'Now I feel that I'm getting it in my old age. I notice it every two weeks or so . . . I'm not sure what it is. Gloom because of the way life is? Every once in a while it hits me.' His wife knows what to do. 'Let me be very honest about it:

when he turns quiet and sombre, I stroke him and then we end up making love together, and things are good again.'[15]

So in elderly emigrants the associations of the present time bite at the oldest of memories like a snake biting its own tail. It might be the smell of new milk or freshly mown grass, the rattle of a door, the image of a brick path glistening in the rain. However perceived, these associations lead to something they saw or experienced as children: faces, their own former neighbourhoods, voices. It is as if contact is made in their memories between opposite poles in time, and through that contact nostalgia is recharged, reviving the suffering that was so intense in their first years abroad but seemed to ebb away after that. In emigrants the normal symptoms of old age seem to conspire to arouse nostalgia. And it is not only reminiscences that play tricks on them. The language they acquired, even if they have been speaking it daily for fifty years, starts to wear thin in places and their mother tongue shows through. Some dream in Frisian again for the first time, and in those dreams they have their own names once more. Shirley dreams as Sjoerdje, Hetty as Hendrikje. Dave is Douwe again in his dreams and realizes when he wakes that there is no one left alive who will ever call him Doutsje.

But the real nostalgia factory is time, which makes emigrants of us all. In old age you reach the conclusion that, without putting in an application, without so much as noticing, you have been dispatched by an emigration agency. Even if you have stayed right where you were, growing old in the midst of familiar things, your reminiscences impress upon you that you are no longer living in the land of your youth. You find yourself in a foreign country without ever having left. Thinking back to those early days forces you to conclude that there are many things now that exist only in your memory.

Notes

Preface

1. S. van den Oord, *Eeuwelingen. Levensverhalen van honderdjarigen in Nederland*, Contact, Amsterdam, 2002, p. 106.
2. C. Dickens, *A Tale of Two Cities*, London, 1859, bk. 3, ch. 9 'The game made'.
3. G. Grass, *Peeling the Onion*, Harvill Secker, London, 2007.
4. 'Günter Grass im Interview', *Frankfurter Allgemeine Zeitung*, 12 August 2006.
5. H. Speerstra, *Cruel Paradise. Life stories of Dutch emigrants*, trans. H. Baron, Eerdmans, Grand Rapids, MI, 2005. This is an abridged version of a book first published in Frisian, the second language of the Netherlands, called *It wrede paradys. Libbensferhalen fan Fryske folksferhuzers* (Friese Pers Boekerij, Leeuwarden, 1999). The book also appeared in Dutch, in a version translated and adapted by the author, called *Het wrede paradijs. Het levensverhaal van de emigrant*, Contact, Amsterdam, 2000. The quotations included in this book come directly from the English version if they are included in it, and have otherwise been translated from the original Frisian version, or in one case from the Dutch version, since it occurs only there.

1 The longest stage

1. P. Thane (ed.), *The Long History of Old Age*, Thames and Hudson, London, 2005.
2. D. Draaisma, 'A ship, gradually lowering sail', *Nature* 439 (2006), pp. 663–4.
3. K. Hazelzet, *De levenstrap*, Uitgeverij Catena, Zwolle, 1994.
4. A. Janssen, *Grijsaards in zwart-wit. De verbeelding van de ouderdom in de Nederlandse prentkunst (1550–1650)*, Walburg Pers, Zutphen, 2007.

2 Forgetful

1. M.A. McDaniel & G.O. Einstein, *Prospective Memory. An overview and synthesis of an emerging field*, Sage, Thousand Oaks, CA, 2007.
2. M.J. Guynn, M.A. McDaniel & G.O. Einstein, 'Prospective memory: When reminders fail', *Memory & Cognition* 26:2 (1998), pp. 287–98.
3. M. Izaute, P. Chambres & S. Larochelle, 'Feeling-of-knowing for proper names', *Canadian Journal of Experimental Psychology* 56:4 (2002), pp. 263–72.
4. P.G. Rendell, A.D. Castel & F.I.M. Craik, 'Memory for proper names in old age: A disproportionate impairment?' *Quarterly Journal of Experimental Psychology* 58A:1 (2005), pp. 54–71.
5. G. Cohen & D.M. Burke, 'Memory for proper names: A review', *Memory* 1:4 (1993), pp. 249–63.
6. M. Milders, B. Deelman & I. Berg, 'Rehabilitation of memory for people's names', *Memory* 6:1 (1998), pp. 21–36.
7. G.D. Gaskell, D.B. Wright & C.A. O'Muircheartaigh, 'Telescoping of landmark events', *Public Opinion Quarterly* 64 (2000), pp. 77–89.
8. N.R. Brown, L.J. Rips & S.K. Shevell, 'Subjective dates of natural events in very long term memory', *Cognitive Psychology* 17 (1985), pp. 139–77.
9. R.W.H.M. Ponds, *Forgetfulness and Cognitive Aging*, PhD thesis, Maastricht University, 1998.
10. I.W. Schmidt, I.J. Berg & B.G. Deelman, 'Illusory superiority in self-reported memory of older adults', *Aging, Neuropsychology, and Cognition* 6 (2000), pp. 288–301.
11. P. Rabbitt & V. Abson, 'Lost and found: Some logical and methodological limitations of self-report questionnaires as tools to study cognitive ageing', *British Journal of Psychology* 81 (1990), pp. 1–16.
12. R.W.H.M. Ponds & J. Jolles, 'Memory complaints in elderly people: The role of memory abilities, metamemory, depression, and personality', *Educational Gerontology* 22 (1996), pp. 341–57.

13. K. van het Reve, *Ik heb nooit iets gelezen*, G. A. van Oorschot, Amsterdam, 2003, p. 349.

3 The forgetfulness market

1. E. Tulving, 'Are there 256 different kinds of memory?', in J.S. Nairne (ed.), *The Foundations of Remembering. Essays in honor of Henry L. Roediger, III*, Psychology Press, New York, 2007, pp. 39–51.

2. J. van Loon & B. Ros, 'Oeps, vergeten!', *Zin* 3 (2007), pp. 40–4.

3. R.W.H.M. Ponds & F. Verhey, *Geheugensteun*, Kosmos-Z&K Uitgevers, Utrecht, 2000.

4. D. Draaisma, *Why Life Speeds Up As You Get Older*, Cambridge University Press, Cambridge, 2012, p. 102.

5. B.L. Beyerstein, 'Whence cometh the myth that we only use 10% of our brains?', in S. Della Sala (ed.), *Mind Myths. Exploring popular assumptions about the mind and brain*, Wiley, Chichester, 1999, pp. 3–24.

6. K.L. Higbee & S.L. Clay, 'College students' beliefs in the ten-percent myth', *Journal of Psychology* 132:5 (1998), pp. 469–76.

7. A. Winter & R. Winter, *Build Your Brain Power*, St Martin's Press, London, 1986; S. Witt, *How to be Twice as Smart*, Simon & Schuster, New York, 1983; D.V. Lewis, *How to Master Your Memory*, Gulf Publishing, Houston, TX, 1962, p. 4; S. Ostrander, L. Schroeder & N. Ostrander, *Superlearning*, Dell, New York, 1979, p. 15; C. Rose, *Accelerated Learning*, Dell, New York, 1987, p. 4; M. Adetumbi, *You're a Better Student Than You Think*, Adex, Huntsville, AL, 1992, p. 11.

8. A. Battro, *Half a Brain is Enough*, Cambridge University Press, Cambridge, 2000.

9. D.J. Herrmann & M.M. Gruneberg, *Verbeter uw geheugen. Technieken om vergeetachtigheid te verhelpen, het geheugen aan te scherpen en de mentale fitheid te verbeteren*, Deltas, Aartselaar, 2002, p. 108.

10. D. O'Brien, *How to Develop a Perfect Memory*, Pavilion Books, London, 1993, p. 90.

11. F.C.J. Stevens, C.D. Kaplan, R.W.H.M. Ponds & J. Jolles, 'The importance of active lifestyles for personal memory performance and memory self-knowledge', *Basic and Applied Social Psychology* 23:2 (2001), pp. 137–45.

12. L.G. Hodgson & S.J. Cutler, 'Looking for signs of Alzheimer's disease', *International Journal of Aging and Human Development* 56:4 (2003), pp. 323–43.

13. Ponds & Verhey, *Geheugensteun*.

4 Reminiscences

1. R. Chirbes, *Los disparos del cazador*, Editorial Anagrama, Barcelona, 1994.
2. Chirbes, *Los disparos*, p. 65.
3. D. Draaisma, 'De zin van reminiscenties', *Tijdschrift voor Gerontologie en Geriatrie* 35 (2004), pp. 139–42.
4. A. Jansari & A.J. Parkin, 'Things that go bump in your life: Explaining the reminiscence bump in autobiographical memory', *Psychology and Aging* 11 (1996), pp. 85–91.
5. J.M. Fitzgerald, 'Autobiographical memory and conceptualizations of the self', in M.A. Conway, D.C. Rubin, H. Spinnler & W.A. Wagenaar (eds.), *Theoretical Perspectives on Autobiographical Memory*, Kluwer, Dordrecht, 1992, pp. 99–114.
6. D. Draaisma, *Why Life Speeds Up As You Get Older. How memory shapes our past*, Cambridge University Press, Cambridge, 2006.
7. G. Grass, *Peeling the Onion*, Harvill Secker, London, 2007.
8. N.L. Mergler & M.D. Goldstein, 'Why are there old people? Senescence as biological and cultural preparedness for the transmission of information', *Human Development* 26 (1983), pp. 72–90.
9. R.W. Schrauf & D.C. Rubin, 'Bilingual autobiographical memory in older adult immigrants: A test of cognitive explanations of the reminiscence bump and the linguistic encoding of memories', *Journal of Memory and Language* 39 (1998), pp. 437–57.
10. J.B. Charles, *Volg het spoor terug*, De Bezige Bij, Amsterdam, 1953.
11. M. Dijkgraaf & M. Meijer, *Het beslissende boek. Nederlandse en Vlaamse schrijvers over het boek dat hun leven veranderde*, Uitgeverij Prometheus, Amsterdam, 2002, p. 68.
12. Ibid., p. 118.
13. Ibid., p. 142.
14. Ibid., p. 143.
15. S.F. Larsen, 'Memorable books: Recall of reading and its personal context', in R.J. Kreuz & M.S. MacNealy (eds.), *Empirical Approaches to Literature and Aesthetics*, Ablex, Norwood, NJ, 1996, pp. 583–99.
16. M.B. Holbrook & R.M. Schindler, 'Some exploratory findings on the development of musical tastes', *Journal of Consumer Research* 16 (1989), pp. 119–24.
17. H. Schuman, R.F. Belli & K. Bischoping, 'The generational basis of historical knowledge', in J.W. Pennebaker, D. Paez & B. Rime (eds.), *Collective Memories of Political Events*, Erlbaum, Mahwah, NJ, 1997, pp. 47–77.

18. J.R. Sehulster, 'In my era: Evidence for the perception of a special period of the past', *Memory* 4 (1996), pp. 145–58.
19. W.R. Mackavey, J.E. Malley & A.J. Steward, 'Remembering autobiographically consequential experiences: Content analysis of psychologists' accounts of their lives', *Psychology and Aging* 6:1 (1991), pp. 50–9.
20. D. Pillemer, 'Momentous events and the life story', *Review of General Psychology* 5:2 (2001), pp. 123–34.
21. D. Berntsen & D.C. Rubin, 'Emotionally charged autobiographical memories across the life span: The recall of happy, sad, traumatic, and involuntary memories', *Psychology and Aging* 17:4 (2002), pp. 636–52.
22. S.M.J. Janssen, *Events in Memory and Environment*, PhD thesis, University of Amsterdam, 2007.
23. P. Costa & R. Kastenbaum, 'Some aspects of memories and ambitions in centenarians', *Journal of Genetic Psychology* 110 (1967), pp. 3–16.
24. P. Fromholt, D.B. Mortensen, P. Torpdahl, L. Bender, P. Larsen & D.C. Rubin, 'Life-narrative and word-cued autobiographical memories in centenarians: Comparisons with 80-year-old control, depressed, and dementia groups', *Memory* 11:1 (2003), pp. 81–8.
25. S. van den Oord, *Eeuwelingen. Levensverhalen van honderdjarigen in Nederland*, Contact, Amsterdam, 2002.
26. Ibid., p. 118.
27. Ibid., p. 77.
28. Ibid., p. 15.
29. Ibid., p. 163.
30. Ibid., p. 206.
31. Ibid., p. 297.
32. Ibid., p. 207.
33. Ibid., p. 100.
34. Ibid., p. 207.
35. Ibid., p. 110.
36. Ibid., p. 256.
37. Ibid., p. 286.
38. Ibid., p. 231.

5 The joy of calling up memories

1. Aristotle, *Rhetoric*, trans. W. Rhys Roberts, Clarendon Press, Oxford, 1924, bk. 2, ch. 13.
2. Ibid., bk. 2, ch. 12.
3. Ibid., bk. 2, ch. 14.

4. M. Frisch, *Tagebuch 1966–1971*, Suhrkamp, Frankfurt, 1979, p. 137. Frisch wrote about the Voluntary Death Society in his journals and elsewhere. *Tagebuch 1966–1971* is available in English (*Sketchbook 1966–1971*, Harcourt Brace Jovanovich, New York, 1974) but quotations in this edition have been translated from the original German editions of *Tagebuch 1966–1971* and the *Gesammelte Werke*.
5. Frisch, *Tagebuch 1966–1971*, p. 134.
6. Ibid., p. 96.
7. Ibid., p. 99.
8. Ibid., p.102.
9. M. Frisch, *Gesammelte Werke*, vol. 6.1, Suhrkamp, Frankfurt, 1976, p. 100.
10. Frisch, *Tagebuch 1966–1971*, p. 99.
11. R. Butler, 'The life review: An interpretation of reminiscence in the aged', *Psychiatry* 26:1 (1963), pp. 65–76.
12. P.G. Coleman, 'Erinnerung und Lebensrückblick im höheren Lebensalter', *Zeitschrift für Gerontologie und Geriatrie* 30 (1997), pp. 362–7.
13. H. Loning, *Geheugen in beeld. In gesprek met historische foto's binnen de reminiscentiemethodiek*, Drents Archief, Assen, 2004.

6 The good son

1. O. Sacks, 'A symposium on memory', *Threepenny Review* 100 (Winter 2005), p. 20.
2. O. Sacks, *Uncle Tungsten. Memories of a chemical boyhood*, Alfred A. Knopf, New York, 2001, p. 134.
3. Ibid., p. 13.
4. Ibid., p. 23.
5. Ibid., pp. 23–4.
6. Ibid., p. 24.

7 Wisdom in hindsight

1. N. Matsier, *Gesloten huis*, De Bezige Bij, Amsterdam, 1994, p. 30.
2. W. Willems, *Stadskind*, Bert Bakker, Amsterdam, 2003, p. 27.
3. Grass, *Peeling the Onion*, Harvill Secker, London, 2007, pp. 29–30.
4. Ibid., p. 160.
5. Ibid., p. 13.
6. Ibid., p. 16.

7. Ibid., p. 18.
8. D.S. Woodruff & J.E. Birren, 'Age changes and cohort differences in personality', *Developmental Psychology* 6:2 (1972), pp. 252–9.
9. D. Offer, *The Psychological World of the Teenager*, Basic Books, New York, 1969; D. Offer & J.B. Offer, *From Teenage to Young Manhood. A psychological study*, Basic Books, New York, 1975.
10. D. Offer, M. Kaiz, K.I. Howard & E.S. Bennett, 'The altering of reported experiences', *Journal of American Academy of Child and Adolescent Psychiatry* 39 (2000), pp. 735–42.

8 The nostalgia factory

1. H. Speerstra, *Cruel Paradise. Life stories of Dutch emigrants*, trans. H. Baron, Eerdmans, Grand Rapids, MI, 2005.
2. Ibid., p. 161.
3. Speerstra, *Het wrede paradijs. Het levensverhaal van de emigrant*, Contact, Amsterdam, 2000, p. 50.
4. Speerstra, *Cruel Paradise*, pp. 32–3.
5. Ibid., p. 194.
6. J. Lindner, *Heimwee. Een pathopsychologisch onderzoek*, H.J. Paris, Amsterdam, 1941; J. Bergsma, *Militair heimwee*, unpublished PhD thesis, Groningen University, 1963.
7. A.D. Ritivoi, *Yesterday's Self. Nostalgia and the immigrant identity*, Rowman & Littlefield, Lanham, MD, 2002.
8. Ibid., p. 19.
9. P. van Albada, 'The past is a foreign country: Een korte geschiedenis van de heimweeziekte', in M. Baudet & R. Steenbergen (eds.), *Heimwee. Een anatomie van het verlangen naar elders*, Balans, Amsterdam, 2004, pp. 23–32.
10. K. Jaspers, *Heimweh und Verbrechen*, F.C.W. Fogel, Leipzig, 1909.
11. A.J. van Vliet, *Homesickness. Antecedents, consequences and mediating processes*, Ponsens & Looijen, Wageningen, 2001.
12. M.A.L. van Tilburg, *When it Hurts to Leave Home. Meaning, manifestations and management of homesickness*, unpublished PhD thesis, Tilburg University, 1998.
13. Cited in Ritivoi, *Yesterday's Self*, p. 24.
14. Speerstra, *It wrede paradys. Libbensferhalen fan Fryske folksferhuzers*, Friese Pers Boekerij, Leeuwarden, 1999, pp. 302–3.
15. Speerstra, *Cruel Paradise*, p. 185.

Acknowledgments

Figure 1 on page 9 depicting the 'Ages of Man' is *Die Lebenstreppe* (Haarlem, seventeenth-century), held in the collection of the Museum Kurhaus Kleve, Germany. © Museum Kurhaus Kleve (Photography: Annegret Gossens). Figure 2 on page 59 is from P. Fromholt, D.B. Mortensen, P. Torpdahl, L. Bender, P. Larsen & D.C. Rubin, 'Life-narrative and word-cued autobiographical memories in centenarians: Comparisons with 80-year-old control, depressed, and dementia groups', *Memory* 11:1 (2003), pp. 81–8. Figure 3 on page 69 is from *NRC Handelsblad*, 21 June 2008, Yassine Salihine/University of Groningen. Both graphs have been redrawn by Martin Brown. Figure 4 on page 96 of a family of peat-cutters in Valthermond (1910–20), taken by R.H. Herwig, is owned by the Drents Museum, Assen, and is reproduced with their permission.

Part of the chapter 'The nostalgia factory' was first published in M. Baudet and R. Steenbergen (eds.), *Heimwee. Een anatomie van het verlangen naar elders*, Uitgeverij Balans, Amsterdam, 2004. A shorter version of the interview with Oliver Sacks appeared on 1 October 2005 in the science and education supplement of *NRC Handelsblad*. On 6 October 2007 that same supplement published an article of which several passages have been adapted for use in the chapter 'Reminiscences'. Extracts from 'The longest stage' appeared in *Nature*, 9 February 2006.

For their comments on the manuscript and for timely words of encouragement I would like to thank Patrick Everard, Rudo Hartman, Gerard Pels and Eva de Valk. Finally, I would like to thank Liz Waters for her elegant translation, and my copy-editor Jenny Roberts. They both wonced miracles on the manuscript and did so with tact and sensitivity.

Index